The Power

11 Ways Women Gain Unhealthy Weight and How You Can Take Charge of Them

Sue Ellin Browder

John Wiley & Sons, Inc.

New York • Chichester • Weinheim • Brisbane • Singapore • Toronto

For my lifelong collaborator, Walter,
who has always known
that all true power
springs from the power of love

Published by John Wiley & Sons, Inc.
Published simultaneously in Canada

This publication is designed to provide accurate and authoritative information in regard to the subject matter covered. It is sold with the understanding that the publisher is not engaged in rendering professional services. If professional advice or other expert assistance is required, the services of a competent professional person should be sought.

Library of Congress Cataloging-in-Publication Data:

Browder, Sue Ellin
The power: 11 ways women gain unhealthy weight
and how you can take charge of them / Sue Ellin Browder
p. cm.
ISBN 0-471-37968-9 (cloth : alk. paper)
1. Weight loss. 2. Overweight women. I. Title

RM222.2 .B7827 2001
613.7'045—dc21   00-047765

Printed in the United States of America

10 9 8 7 6 5 4 3 2 1

Contents

Introduction

Come with me now, and let's go on a quest. It's not a quest for the holy grail, although my agent called this book *The Grail* when it first appeared in her office. But it's a soulful journey nonetheless. We will start out together, but eventually you will go your own way. Because in the end, the journey we're about to take will lead you to a kind of superconfidence, the kind of superconfidence that comes from understanding what you need to take charge of your health.

The journey that led to this book began for me as a medical journalist about seven years ago when magazine editors suddenly began clamoring for stories about weight loss. At first, I eagerly took on the assignments, because I too have had my weight struggles. I've been a binge eater. I've been off and on probably hundreds of diets. Basically, I "dieted," if you could call it that, almost constantly between the ages of twelve and fifty-one.

Because of my own struggles, I pursued these assignments with an unbridled passion, and my enthusiasm apparently showed. My *Woman's Day* article "Can Diet Pills Make You Thin?"—which warned against the overprescribing of fen-phen long before that particular drug combination killed some women—was so thorough and balanced that M.D.'s from all over the United States asked permission to photocopy the story and hand it out to their patients. "How to Flatten Your Stomach," the *Reader's Digest*'s lead story of June 1995, was also popular—so much so that the next year the editor in chief commissioned me to do a repeat. That's when I did "Flatten Your Tummy—Forever," written from the angle of "how weight-loss winners do it." I did a number of other weight-loss stories, including "Dieting Online" and "Diet Traps." The second ran first in *Woman's Day* and was then picked up by both *Reader's Digest* and a "life-enrichment" magazine called *Personal Excellence,* where it ran alongside pieces by gurus like Deepak Chopra, Stephen R. Covey, and the Dalai Lama. Quite inadvertently, I had become the "diet guru" of the magazines.

There was only one problem. I had amassed so much research by that point, I knew that many weight-loss "truisms" in our society are dead wrong. Are overweight women fat simply because they eat too many calories? Does exercise help everybody lose weight? Does dieting save all overweight women's lives? Most people would answer these questions with an unequivocal yes. But many top weight-loss researchers are answering these same questions with a resounding no—and they are now being hotly debated.

Just as suddenly as I began writing diet articles, I found myself having to turn down diet assignments. When one bright young editor phoned to request a huge two-part article on exercise and dieting (a plum, considering I had all the research done), I had to say no, explaining that I believed the old-hat ideas she wanted to include were misleading to women. Instead of asking me why, she breezily observed she'd just assign the story to somebody else.

After I hung up the phone, I sat alone in my office. I stared at my four-drawer file cabinets, now overflowing with medical research revealing the real truths about weight loss. I thought back to the many women I'd met online who were still fat and desperately searching for answers. These women wanted—and dearly needed—access to the latest and most reliable research, so they could apply it intelligently to their own lives. Their need was more than cosmetic. For some, getting accurate information was a matter of life or death. I also recalled those amazing women who'd beaten the odds. When I added my own interviews to the medical reports I'd collected about these women, I had information on more than three thousand weight-loss winners.

Sitting alone in my office that October day, a chilling realization suddenly hit me: no doctor was going to write this book. Six years had passed since an eminent endocrinologist had first told me there were many ways to be fat. Yet no one had told women the many new answers about fat that were already in the medical literature. Eventually the truth would get out, but it might take another ten years—or longer. Meanwhile, women were struggling to take charge of their health in a sea of misinformation. Women couldn't wait another ten years. They needed this information right now.

I heaved a heavy sigh of responsibility. I knew from my past experiences with writing books it would be two, maybe even three years before I'd have my life back. Still, it's a journalist's job to get out the truth. If we don't do it, who will? I took a long, slow sip from my cup of coffee, clicked on my computer, and began the outline for *The Power*.

It is likely that you haven't discovered the secret to successful weight control. You may have tried dozens of diets, sought help from doctors, psychiatrists, hypnotists, personal trainers, and gurus—all to no avail. Perhaps your focus has been so completely trained on the "ideal" that you have been unable to see the obvious solution: a plan of action that is personalized to fit you, not a passing cultural fad.

—C. Wayne Callaway, M.D.
George Washington University

PART ONE

Embrace Your Individuality

CHAPTER 1

The Weight-Loss Winners

Once in a blue moon, you meet a woman like Gwen. She doesn't merely have high self-esteem. She has an unbridled *superconfidence* that helps her bounce back quickly from defeat. When she and her best friend Sara were fired from their personnel jobs in the aerospace industry, Sara said, "I'm ruined. I'll never find work. I was an idiot to stay in that job for so long." Meanwhile, Gwen told herself, "Hey, it's true our company was downsizing. But I'm a brilliant people person, and I can find plenty of work if I'll just shift directions." Within a month, Gwen landed a new job as a travel agent and was soon selling more cruises than anyone in her office; meanwhile, Sara was still sending out résumés, counting the days until her unemployment checks stopped.

Gwen's gung ho attitude doesn't vanish when she leaves the office: it permeates her whole life. When her boyfriend insisted he needed space to date other women, did she spend months fretting that she was unlovable and wondering where she went wrong? Not Gwen. "He's got some real issues he needs to work out," she matter-of-factly explained. "He'll be back when he realizes the huge mistake he's made. Meanwhile, I'm not sitting around by the phone. I'm going to get out and have fun!" When she tells a joke at a party and nobody laughs, does she spend the rest of the night silently berating herself for looking foolish? No, she blames the *joke*: "Okay, so that was a real groaner. Here's a better one." And soon she has everyone within earshot giggling along *with* her.

Now here's a secret only a few people know (I didn't know it myself until recently): Gwen used to be fat. In fact, she once weighed over 250 pounds. She now weighs 121 pounds and has been at that weight for years. One of the winners I found and interviewed after reading studies about more than three thousand of these women, Gwen and others like her have convinced me that the superconfidence you need to take charge of your weight isn't an inborn talent only a few lucky women possess: it's an ability any of us can develop. Unflappable self-confidence regarding your weight is a skill you can learn. What's more, the latest research coming out of university medical center labs reveals this skill may do far more than help you resist fattening foods. It may affect your biology right down to the level of the fat cell. Superconfidence can help you find your healthy weight not just for a few months, but for life.

As its title implies, this book is not about "dieting" in the obsolete sense that you're given only one rigid prescription, telling you exactly what to eat and how much to exercise. Rather, this book will give you all the skills you need to match the latest information about weight control to your own individual way of being overweight, to create the plan that is right for you. In a world of constant change, overly rigid, "single-magic-bullet" diet prescriptions are now being discarded. Why? Because real women are much too diverse to be so narrowly pigeonholed. You require and deserve more.

A Need for Change

Unfortunately, those who persist in trying to apply overly narrow single-magic-bullet prescriptions across the board to diverse groups of overweight women only sap your confidence and create more confusion. If you're still stressed about your weight, perhaps after years of searching for answers, you're hardly alone. When one hundred people were asked to choose their most frequent daily hassles from a list of 117 irritating, frustrating, and distressing demands, "concerns about weight" were number one, way above worries about taxes, crime, inflation, problems with coworkers, or even having too much to do.

The main reason women are still so stressed about weight is that we're continually told how important it is for our health, yet we're never given all the information we need to take charge. We lack confidence largely because we're never told all the facts. This book will give you the straight talk about women's weight: what's known, what's not known, how it applies to you, and how strong, independent women can become scientists of their own bodies and at last find answers that work. As a medical writer and an ordinary woman like you who has had my own weight struggles, I have no pet theories to promote, no academic turf to defend, no clinic to fund. This book emerged solely because I was curious and honestly trying to learn the truth about weight control; and once I did find the truth (which turned out to be even more intriguing than I'd thought it would be), I had to tell you about it. It was just too important for women to know.

Women need the superconfidence to take charge because weight research is changing dramatically. In fact, we're currently caught up in one of the most fascinating paradigm shifts to hit weight-control science in the past 150 years. Since the 1960s, more than two hundred thousand studies and articles about obesity and weight gain have been published in prestigious peer-reviewed medical journals in North America and Europe. Major international conferences on obesity have been held in cities around the globe, including New York City, Berlin, Jerusalem, Toronto, Paris, Rome, and Kobe, Japan. Millions, if not billions, of dollars have been poured into research to determine why we gain weight and what fat means to our health. Now that 25 to 35 percent of people in Western industrialized societies are overweight, we have witnessed a global assault on this global problem.

So the question is, What's been the result of all this time, effort, and money? The answer: a breakthrough understanding of weight control is emerging. Some fat is now seen as healthy. Other fat is unhealthy, but now known to be caused by far more than just eating too much and exercising too little. In this new, much broader understanding, unhealthy fat is seen as many different conditions that spring from many biological, psychological, and cultural causes, including stress, depression, anger, past sexual abuse, smoking, too much alcohol, social injustice, fat-promoting medications and surgeries, excess dieting, hormones, and genes. These conditions can and, in fact, must be approached in different ways. When the dust from this new understanding settles, almost nothing you have been taught to believe about fat and your health will ever again be the same. Eat less, exercise more, while it's not going down the tubes entirely as a prescription, was never good enough—certainly never *enough*—to help most of us find our healthiest weights. There are many ways to be fat (and we'll discuss them all), but stress plays a much bigger role than we've ever been told. Before you've read even half of this book, you'll know why a healthy weight is a happy weight and why becoming superconfident can not only help you lose fat but also help you live longer.

But, first, let's start with a story.

The Mystery

It was a warm, sensuous spring day at the University of Missouri in Columbia, the kind of day that makes people feel like starting fresh in their lives. A bunch of us, all college women, were in a dorm sitting cross-legged on the floor playing poker, when two friends challenged each other to see who could lose 30 pounds faster. "We're going to do it—yeah!!! I'm going to beat your butt!" Becca cheered, slapping her cards down. "That's a full house!" The rest of us joined the camaraderie by betting who would win. Since Becca and Melissa were both twenty-one and roommates, ate in the same cafeteria, and even took the same PE class together, the contest looked like a toss-up. I bet five bucks on Melissa.

Weeks passed, then months. Becca looked slimmer and slimmer. All smiles, she kept buying new clothes because the old ones no longer fit. Melissa, on the other hand, kept losing weight, but gaining it back. Once a week on Saturdays—her self-proclaimed "pig-out day"—Becca ate whatever she pleased. Poor Melissa, after surviving on nothing but cottage cheese and fruit for a week, would eat one piece of pizza and regain two pounds. By summer break, Becca was proclaimed the hands-down winner. She went home superconfident and 30 pounds lighter. Melissa went home fat and cranky: she'd lost 17 pounds—and gained them all back.

The memory of that contest, which turned out to be no contest, has stayed with me for close to thirty years. At the time of our poker game, I was an investigative journalist in training and learning to take nothing at face value. There was no way then to explain how Becca and Melissa could have gone on exactly the same diet, done exactly the same exercise, and yet gotten such drastically different results. So I figured Melissa must have secretly cheated. I envisioned her sneaking out of the dorm late at night to scarf down hot-fudge sundaes and cookies while the rest of us slept.

Now I know better. I now know it's quite common for two women of exactly the same age, weight, and height to go on exactly the same diet and get totally opposite results. Overweight women vary dramatically in their responses to different diets because they vary dramatically in their ways to be fat.

Think of it this way. Medical science has cured smallpox, malaria, and polio and is now hot on the heels of cancer. So why can't it make a fat woman thin? The answer is simple: we've been looking at weight loss all wrong. Like perhaps as many as 10 percent of overweight women, Melissa may have had a seldom-diagnosed hormonal disorder called Polycystic Ovary Syndrome (PCOS), which makes it nearly impossible to lose weight through diet and exercise alone. Or perhaps she had Depression Fat, Anger Fat, Post-Trauma Fat, Medication-Caused Fat, or any of a host of other problems. Melissa always swore she wasn't cheating, and now I'm convinced she was telling the truth. Whatever her problem, it apparently wasn't one of the "environmental obesities" caused simply by eating too much and exercising too little.

Women vary greatly—not only in their ways of being fat, but in their abilities to take control of their health. Some trust only external authorities, in the form of nutritionists, personal trainers, doctors, skinny Hollywood actresses, and other diet gurus. They wait for someone else to provide all the answers. When one rigid, pre-planned diet formula fails them, they either give up or try another. They distrust themselves, have no faith in their abilities, are quick to despair—and usually stay fat. At the other extreme are those enterprising, superconfident women I talked to in the course of writing this book, the weight-control winners. Long before scientists discovered there are many ways to be fat, these women intuitively found their own paths. Some are happy and fat, knowing they're healthy. They know that virtue and beauty come from within and respect their large, healthy bodies. Other winners were once fat and on their way to heart attacks or diabetes but have slimmed down and are now keeping the weight off. Superconfident winners have a deep-rooted faith in their own instincts and refuse to accept defeat—like one tenacious woman who invented twenty different diets for herself before she finally designed one that worked. She and other winners have taught me that women can—and do—lose weight permanently. How? A superconfident woman named Alia put it well: "It's not a matter of willpower, but power."

This book is a guide to such power. Along with the new paradigm of weight control and the many ways to be fat, you will learn about the superconfidence of the weight-control winners, why they succeed where others fail. If you are fat and healthy, the changes we're about to discuss will help you transcend negative societal messages and learn to trust your large body. If you have unhealthy fat, the principles I've learned from the winners will help you choose the best options for you and then muster the faith in yourself to follow them.

I also hope this book will empower you to find a doctor who will treat you as an equal partner in your own healing. Even with the new understandings about fat, the answers aren't simple. But doctors must remember that you have a very special knowledge that can be a font of healing wisdom: the knowledge you've gained from a lifetime of living in your own body. Trust your feelings. If you know why you've gained weight and your doctor refuses to listen, find another doctor.

The weight-control winners I talked to have traveled a long distance, and they have something to show you. They're not here to teach you how to be just like them. They're here to teach you how to become more deeply yourself.

Throughout history, women have woven supportive networks from their common needs and shared experiences. Whenever you find women facing life's crises—birth, death, illness, troubles with love or work—you usually find other women there, helping. You might think of this book as an old-fashioned sewing circle or quilting bee, a comfortable place where women have banded together to tell their healing stories.

CHAPTER 2

One Size Does Not Fit All

I can evade questions without help. What I need is answers.

—John F. Kennedy

Maggie hated her high-pressure sales job, smoked two packs of cig-arettes a day, drank gallons of coffee to stay alert, wound down in the evenings with a few glasses of wine, slept poorly, and never took a day off. One day, when she stepped on the scale in her doctor's office, she weighed 192 pounds. The doctor told her, "Your blood pressure is exorbitant. If you don't lose weight, you'll die." He handed her a diet typed on a green piece of paper. The diet listed exactly what foods and how much she should eat for each meal of the week. Nothing could look simpler—nor be harder. At home, Maggie followed the diet to a tee and starved herself for three months. Hard as it was, every evening she cooked two meals: one for her, one for her family. Her stress levels mounted. Her head-aches got worse. Her insecurity skyrocketed. When she returned for a follow-up visit, the doctor coldly studied her chart. Then he said, "You've lost only two pounds. You've been cheating."

At that moment, Maggie looked at her doctor, and something in her just clicked. She realized this doctor, self-assured as he looked, had no real answers for her. If she was ever going to heal, she would have to take charge. Furious and exhausted from stress and starva-tion, Maggie went home and designed her own eating plan, one that didn't require cooking two dinners. She also quit smoking, traded her coffee for herbal tea, and began addressing the stress that triggered her binges. She learned to meditate and took up yoga. She quit her stressful sales job and started a home pet-sitting service. In eight months, she'd lost 62 pounds.

Thinking she'd teach her doctor a lesson that might help other women, Maggie went back to him for her annual exam. The doctor examined her forms, not even looking in her direction. "Your blood pressure is normal, and I see you've finally taken my advice and lost weight—about time," he said. Then before she could tell him it was no thanks to his diet, he picked up his clipboard and disappeared out the door. Vowing that very second to find a new doctor, Maggie checked her watch: her annual physical had lasted just seven minutes.

Is it any wonder that many doctors never hear inspiring weight-loss success stories like Maggie's? Such self-cures seldom get reported in the medical literature because women who find the confidence to take charge of their weight don't usually tell doctors their biggest secret: I did it my way.

Doing it *your* way is the only answer because you're a unique individual with a unique mind and body. For centuries, physicians and patients alike have been on a quest for the one perfect way to cure excess fat—one solution for this one condition. But excess fat isn't just one condition. Thoughtful scientists have long observed that fat is many different disorders requiring many different solutions. In her book *The Importance of Overweight*, published in 1957, the distinguished eating-disorders specialist Dr. Hilde Bruch wrote: "The current tendency to lump all cases of simple obesity together is at about the same level of scientific exactness that prevailed in medicine when 'a fever' and 'a headache' were considered adequate diagnoses. It is generally known now that fevers and headaches are only symptoms of a great variety of disorders. In our approach to 'overweight' we still act like the old-time physician who put his hand on a patient and, finding his skin warm, would solemnly pronounce that he suffered from 'a fever' and would proceed to bleed, purge, or starve him."

Behind closed doors in major medical conferences, careful scientists have been discussing *the obesities* (plural) and their various treatments for at least the last quarter century. Since 1975, a number of international medical conferences about body weight have been held in Germany. These prestigious Dahlem Workshops, held at the Free University of Berlin, tend to attract the most knowledgeable obesity experts from around the world. In a 1976 Dahlem

Workshop, half the sessions were devoted in part to the then "new" understanding that excess weight is many syndromes with many different solutions. In a 1997 issue of the prestigious *British Medical Bulletin*, a Cambridge researcher notes, "Obesity is not a single disorder but a heterogeneous group of conditions with multiple causes." In a December 1995 issue of *American Journal of Medicine and Science*, a doctor from the Centers for Disease Control and Prevention in Atlanta writes of the "heterogeneous nature of obesity," noting that only certain types of excess weight (not all of them) put women at increased risk for disease. Other fat is quite healthy. In short, the fact that there are many different ways to be fat, only some of which are unhealthy, isn't just a wild theory: it's common medical knowledge.

Yet despite the insights of these eminent physicians, most of medical science and the popular media persist in viewing fat as a single "problem" with a single solution (eat less, exercise more). We're given sweeping statements like "diets don't work," when in fact they *do* work for some women, but not for others. We're told fat kills, when in fact only *some* ways of being fat increase the risks of disease. Other ways of being fat are perfectly healthy. Is a low-fat diet the right one for you? That depends on you, your body, and why you got fat. The time has come to recognize that not all overweight women are the same, nor do they all have the same problem. If women who need to lose fat and keep it off are ever to become empowered enough to get the job done, these differences cannot be ignored.

The Diet Wars:
A Report from the Front

Several years ago, when a national magazine assigned me to write a cover story called "Flatten Your Tummy," I was delighted to take on the assignment. I wasn't officially "obese" (20 percent or more over my ideal weight), but I wasn't pencil-thin, either. For years, I'd battled an extra 10 pounds . . . then 15 . . . then 20. I'd read every diet book and article on the planet, and all the sensible ones had been versions of exactly the same advice: eat less, exercise more. Now at last, I was going to get paid to ask questions I'd always been burning to ask: What's the very best way to lose weight? What do the experts know that the rest of us don't?

As an investigative medical reporter I'd written stories on everything from fibroids and breast cancer to female heart disease and deadly doctors. So I knew that what passes for popular wisdom in the media seldom completely pans out when you talk to research scientists in their labs. There are always fascinating new developments that haven't been fully reported. But I wasn't prepared for the uproar I was about to encounter.

When I started calling weight-loss researchers and clinicians at Tufts, Yale, Harvard, UCLA, Stanford, and other leading universities, I ran into disagreement over every question I asked. The most distinguished scientists could not agree on how fat we should be, how to measure fat, whether aerobic exercise will flatten your tummy better than weight lifting, how much exercise we need to stay healthy, or even whether diets work.

I asked two leading obesity researchers what seemed to me like a fairly simple, straightforward question: Is there such a thing as a female fat cell (as nutritionist Debra Waterhouse had claimed in her book *Outsmarting the Female Fat Cell*)? In other words, are women's fat cells bigger and more diet-resistant than men's? When I posed this question, I got a no from Jules Hirsch, the dean of obesity research at Rockefeller University, and a yes from George A. Bray, former director of the Pennington Biomedical Research Center at Louisiana State University and the founding editor of the journal *Obesity Research*. Told that Hirsch had said no, Bray replied, "With all respect to my distinguished colleague—he's wrong." I was dumbfounded. If even the nation's leading medical doctors couldn't agree whether a single type of fat cell existed, I thought, is it any wonder ordinary women like me are having so much trouble figuring out how to get and stay thin?

Many scientists still insisted weight gain is simply a matter of too many calories coming in and too few going out. "If you eat too many calories, you'll gain weight—even if you just eat a thousand carrots," declared Gerald Reaven, a highly regarded insulin researcher at Stanford University. That sounded reasonable enough. But other equally reputable doctors insist that eating carbohydrates like those in carrots *cannot* make you fat, even if you ate ten thousand (assuming such a feat could be managed). "What most people don't understand is that the human body literally cannot turn carbohydrates into fat. Rats can turn carbohydrates into fat. But humans can't. It's physiologically impossible," declared one of the biggest guns in obesity research at Harvard University, George Blackburn. Many obesity researchers insisted we should all be on low-fat diets to protect our hearts. Yet Reaven maintained that eating a diet too low in fat can actually increase some people's risk of heart disease. Usually, talking to high-profile scientists clarifies any confusion I have about a medical issue. But in this case, the more authorities I interviewed, the muddier the waters became.

Skinny researchers in Boston were claiming "fat is bad" and that even gaining as little as 10 pounds during one's life could damage the heart. Pudgy researchers in Atlanta and Dallas were saying, "Fat is okay, and diets don't work."

An eating disorders specialist at the University of Cincinnati, Susan Wooley, startled me by insisting that obesity isn't a major health risk for the vast majority of women. Noting that being overweight is actually protective against tuberculosis, osteoporosis, suicide, and lung cancer, she told me: "There is very little evidence that being overweight is more unhealthy than being thin. My argument is this: we know diets don't work very well and there's increasing reason to suspect they may be quite dangerous—so why in the world prescribe them?"

I was stunned. I knew that some pop diets were dangerous, but *all* diets? I soon learned that Wooley had solid evidence to back up her claims.

A study led by Elsie R. Pamuk at the National Center for Chronic Disease Prevention and Health Promotion at the Centers for Disease Control found that going on a diet and succeeding actually *increased* death rates in women (although it reduced them in men). Female dieters in all weight ranges—fat, moderately overweight, and average—who lost 15 percent or more of their weight were two to three times more apt to die from all causes—including heart disease—than women who had lost less than 5 percent of their weight. In other words, female dieters who achieved their goals did not live longer than women who stayed fat. On the contrary, dieting seems to have shortened some women's lives. In a study of 33,760 Iowa women, those who had gained and lost the most weight when they were younger had the highest risk of dying in later life, especially from coronary heart disease. At least six other studies had unearthed variations of this same disturbing finding.

These findings had profound implications for women's health. Yet they had been virtually ignored by the popular press. Why were they overlooked, while studies stressing the dangers of fat and the benefits of dieting continued to be so heavily reported? Should I even be trying to lose weight? Or would losing 15 or 20 pounds actually do me more harm than good? Suppose I had 50 or 100 pounds to lose—then what? Wherever I turned, my questions brought no reassuring answers but only more unsettling questions.

Many of us who've struggled with our weight know well the torments of craving certain foods like brownies or ice cream. But the experts couldn't decide whether these cravings were for carbohydrates or for fat. Nutritional researcher Judith Wurtman made quite a name for herself when she was at MIT by claiming that fat women craved carbohydrates. It was because of some research she did in the late 1980s that the term "carbohydrate craving" was coined. But I soon learned her work had many critics. One of them, Adam Drewnowski, who directs the human nutrition program at the University of Michigan, presented a strong case for the fact that all the foods Wurtman studied—snacks like cookies, cakes, M&M's, and ice cream—weren't actually carbohydrates but combinations of sugar and fat. "What women really crave is fat," he explained. Then he unleashed the ultimate insult one nutrition researcher can hurl at another: "Basically, Judy has been misnaming her foods."

Although I found these endless controversies frustrating as I tried to pull together my story, I also found them compelling. Why? Because from my past experience as a medical reporter, I knew that when intelligent doctors begin passionately squabbling over who's right and who's wrong, that's a clear sign you're at the cutting edge of medical research, a place where something very interesting is about to happen. Heated medical battles like these typically lead not to one side "winning" with the other "losing" but to a whole new understanding of the problem. Once the problem is viewed from a broader, more enlightened perspective, it turns out that good scientists on all sides of the debate were at least partly right. The controversies over salt a few years earlier were a good example. Salt's role—or lack of it—in high blood pressure was hotly debated until it was discovered that some people are "salt-sensitive" and experience a rise in blood pressure in response to even a little extra salt, while others can eat mountains of salt without harm.

Was this same sort of rethinking happening in weight-control research? If so, the changes coming down the pike promised to change our understandings of weight loss completely because the battles weren't taking place in just one or two subspecialty fields: they were being waged everywhere on all fronts.

Many Ways to Be Fat

Finally, one day while talking to George Washington University endocrinologist C. Wayne Callaway, I dropped my "objective journalist" tone for a moment and expressed my frustration. "Here I am trying to write what I thought would be a simple flatten-your-tummy story," I complained. "I've talked to leading experts all over the country. And I can't get a straight answer from anybody!" Immediately pinpointing the trouble, he matter-of-factly replied, "The problem is, there are many ways to be fat. That's the dilemma we all have to struggle with when we put out this information."

I sat in stunned silence for a moment. So many questions in my brain competed to be asked first that I didn't know where to begin. Finally, I just repeated his astonishing words: *Many* ways to be fat? As if the bombshell he'd just dropped were common knowledge, he continued, "Some overweight people, like women with Polycystic Ovary Syndrome, have hormonal imbalances. Others have injuries to their hypothalamus or were sexually abused as kids. Still others really do just eat too much fat or don't exercise enough."

Suddenly, all the heated controversies I'd been hearing over the past two months began to make sense: A new understanding of weight loss truly *was* coming down the pike. In fact, it had already arrived. The passionate scientific arguments I'd been hearing merely reflected the intellectual chaos that frequently accompanies new ideas before a new synthesis emerges.

As I began looking through the medical literature, I found eleven different unhealthy ways to be fat beyond the simple "environmental obesities" (the only kinds of fat that be controlled by diet and exercise alone). What's more, by the doctors' own estimates, these eleven ways to be fat afflict a whopping 85 percent of seriously overweight women.

I also found something else quite surprising: many women who constantly diet in an effort to become superthin have healthy fat. And that includes some who are considerably overweight, according to those ubiquitous weight tables. When women diet to lose this kind of fat, they may do themselves more harm than good.

No responsible doctor would prescribe chemotherapy for a patient without cancer. That would be nonsense. Healthy people should not be given the same treatments as those who are sick. Should a patient with excellent blood pressure take a blood-pressure medication? Of course not. But when it comes to weight, the same diets prescribed for women with *un*healthy fat are given to women who are perfectly healthy.

Does this bizarre practice harm healthy women? Mounting evidence says yes. The most provocative finding so far comes from an American Cancer Society/Centers for Disease Control study of 43,457 women between the ages of forty and sixty-four who had never smoked and were overweight: 28,388 were classified as "healthy"; 15,069 were "unhealthy." For those women in the second group, who actually had fat-related health problems (such as high blood pressure, or a previous history of heart disease, diabetes, or stroke), intentionally trying to lose weight was helpful. Women with unhealthy fat who lost any amount of weight at all—even a few pounds—were 20 percent less apt to die during a thirteen-year period than those who didn't lose weight.

For healthy women, however, it was another story. Those who intentionally tried to lose weight—and succeeded—were 40 to 70 percent more apt to die than fat, healthy women who didn't lose weight.

What's equally disturbing, losing 10 or 15 pounds of healthy fat over and over again (as yo-yo dieters typically do) may even turn it into *unhealthy* fat.

One day, as I was walking along a beach near my home pondering this idea, I suddenly realized the new way the world's most informed scientists are now viewing excess weight parallels a shift that occurred a number of years ago in the field of cancer research. Medical science used to lump all cancers together under one umbrella. When a patient had a malignant tumor, doctors just said she or he had cancer and left it at that. But as research advanced, doctors came to view cancer not just as one disease but as more than a hundred different diseases, all of which need to be treated differently. Even knowing a person has a certain kind of cancer—such as lung cancer—is no longer enough. To determine the right treatment, you also have to know what *kind* of lung cancer it is, whether it's small-cell, squamous cell, large-cell, or something else.

Now a parallel shift has taken place in our understanding of obesity. Scientists used to lump all ways of being overweight in one category—heavy people were just labeled fat or "obese" (a condition thought to be caused simply by eating too much and exercising too little). But now they're recognizing that excess weight isn't just one disease, but *many* disorders with many different causes and many different solutions. Most of the world's most knowledgeable diet doctors, in fact, no longer talk about obesity (singular): they talk about *the obesities*.

The old idea that weight is just a matter of calories in, calories out (or fat in, fat out, if you prefer), is also changing. In real life, weight is, indeed, determined by calories in, calories out, and can be cured "simply" by eating less and exercising more . . . *unless* you happen to be a nonresponder to exercise, *unless* you have a hormonal imbalance, *unless* you're under chronic stress, *unless* you're angry, *unless* you were sexually abused, *unless* you've had your ovaries removed, *unless* you're getting older, *unless* you have a genetic disorder, *unless* you're taking certain medications, *unless, unless, unless.*

In short, trying to treat all the common ways of being overweight with any single prescription would be a lot like trying to cure all fevers with the same prescription, without first considering whether the patient has tuberculosis, the flu, or chicken pox. This analogy is doubly appropriate because some ways of being fat are like TB in that they're potential killers, whereas others are more like chicken pox in that they're usually harmless.

The single-bullet answers worked great for single-cause diseases like smallpox, whooping cough, and polio. When a disorder or disease has only one cause, then it's easy to find one solution. But when it comes to excess fat, which has many *different* causes, one has to find many different solutions.

Lessons from the Rule Breakers

Once I realized this, I became obsessed with finding out everything I could about women's weight. I started collecting articles from medical journals as if they were precious jewels. At first I just had a hundred, then a thousand, then four thousand. I wanted to know everything I could about the many ways to be fat and what to do about them.

I became what my husband, Walter, called "a curious advocate" for overweight women, asking questions any woman would ask if she could only get her doctor to pause long enough to answer them:

- How can I figure out why I'm fat?
- Is my particular type of fat healthy or unhealthy?
- If it's unhealthy, what can I do?
- If it's not damaging my health, how can I make peace with my body and respect its wisdom?

Dishes piled up in the kitchen. Groceries went unpurchased. Here I was writing a book urging women to take charge of their health, and one day I had only coffee and potato chips for breakfast.

As my research progressed, I began noticing many studies that included the phrase "weight-loss maintenance." The most interesting of these studies were of women who'd beaten seemingly impossible odds. They had not only lost weight, they had kept it off. I was fascinated to learn these winners are far more common than we've ever believed. We're frequently told that 85 to 95 percent of women who lose weight eventually regain it all—and then some. But this statistic, I quickly learned, applies only to overweight women who go to university-based diet clinics, where the programs are preplanned by others. Among women who take charge and lose weight *their* way, the victory rate is much higher. Psychologist Stanley Schachter went into Amagansett, a small town on eastern Long Island, and studied a population of ordinary people who had just tried to lose weight on their own. He also interviewed secretaries, grad students, technicians, and professors in his psychology department at Columbia University. Of the people he talked to who'd once been fat, an inspiring 62.5 percent had slimmed down on their own—and *kept* the weight off. What's more, the more overweight they'd been, the greater their success rates were.

The comparison was startling: a 5 to 15 percent success rate for weight clinics, versus a 62.5 percent success rate for people who cure themselves. Women's self-cure rates were *four to twelve times higher* than the cure rates by doctors.

Who were these women? What were their secrets? If weight-control winners were really so common, I figured I should be able to find them myself. It was certainly worth a shot. I started sharing the news about the new paradigm with every woman I met. That's when I discovered a huge "underground" of women who were already using it! They were ahead of their time. Using the new approach to weight control even before doctors had discovered it, these amazing women had taken charge of their health, asked questions, learned everything they could about why they were fat, then intuitively trusted their bodies to help them figure out what to do. Some had healthy fat and were content to stay at their current weight (even if they were quite chubby by societal standards). Others once had unhealthy fat but had ferreted out the cause and then lost it. Many of these women had been at their ideal weights for ten, fifteen, or twenty years. When I told them the news about the many ways to be fat, they confidently replied, "Of course. We knew it all the time." That's when they began to teach me.

Superconfident women know that relying too strongly on any one belief—even such "truisms" as "exercise makes you thin," "calories make you fat," or "all fat is bad"—can prevent us from looking further. By shaping and transforming our thoughts, we free ourselves from their control. In many ways, winners approach their weight-control battles with a freshness similar to that which the Zen masters call the beginner's mind: in the beginner's mind, it is said, there are many possibilities. In the expert's, only a few.

To find out whether you already have the outlook of a winner, ask yourself this question before reading further: If you could take a magic pill right now and lose all the weight you wanted, would you do it? Many people will respond with an immediate, "Yes! Absolutely!"—no ifs, ands, or maybes. Superconfident winners, however, will answer this question with their own questions: "Is the pill safe? How thoroughly has it been tested? How long did the studies last? What are the side effects? Did it work well on women (not men) with my type of fat? How long before I notice results? Will the effects last after I stop? Why this particular pill? Why not another? Why, why, why, why, why?" Women who become winners know the answers may not be simple. But they trust their own abilities to dig out the truth.

Beginning the Journey

As I talked to winners, I felt a transformation in my attitude toward my own weight. A chronic dieter for most of my life, I constantly tried *not* to eat, and I was frequently stressed. For decades, whenever anyone asked me if I wanted a candy bar or a piece of cake, I'd say, "No thanks; I'm on a diet." My husband, Walter, is an extremely tolerant man. But this one habit of mine drove him nuts. Now, to Walter's and my own great relief, I stopped dieting. I started eating whatever I pleased. I stashed my bathroom scale in the back of a closet, where it began to collect dust. To stay relaxed, I began meditating and started going to the beach more often. I went back to church.

I also began paying attention to my body's signals. For the first time in my life, I started to recognize how bad it feels to eat three dozen cookies at a sitting—*before* I'd eaten them. So I'd have a banana instead. My body began telling me when I needed a walk. And, for the first time, I started to listen.

To my astonishment, as my stress over my weight lessened, I began to lose weight. When I'd started the "Flatten Your Tummy" article, I was about 20 pounds above my "ideal." Once I stopped worrying about my weight, 10 of those pounds melted away. Kaput! The day I discovered this (I'd gone to the Y and had stepped on a scale for the first time in months), an immense freedom welled up inside me. After years of dieting, could *not caring* about food be the answer? But then over the next few months, the stress began to mount, my confidence waned, and I felt my jeans getting tighter again. I was really puzzled. What was going on?

Slowly, from talking to winners, I began sorting it out. I came to realize that when we see weight loss as a *goal*, we're looking at it all wrong. Much more often than we've been told, weight is a balancing act between our faith in ourselves, the skills we've developed, and the stressful demands of our lives. Genes and aging count, of course. But within those limits established by nature, how much a woman weighs during any given year tends to reflect how confident and capable she feels. Women who lose weight look extremely confident, and we credit their new figures for their self-assurance. But we have it backward. Winners almost unanimously agree the confidence built on acquired skills comes *first*. They've found not just a better way to eat or exercise but a healthier and truer attitude toward their bodies and themselves. It's this self-awareness, coupled with finding out why they were fat and confidently pursuing their own answers, that ultimately led to their healing.

Women nowadays are often told we need to become medically "empowered" (in the sense we need to take charge of our health). But *power* without valid information is an illusion. How can we make intelligent, effective, *confident* decisions about our weight and our health if we're given only half-truths and never hear all the facts? The answer, of course, is we can't. If today's women still rely too often on external authorities to tell us how much we should weigh and what we should do to get and stay slim, it's only because on some level we know that we still haven't been given all the information we need in this area to become the authors of our own lives.

There's an uneasiness that goes with the severing of one's normal thought patterns about weight, an urge to return to the old, familiar paths one has followed before. But when it comes to the lessons our culture teaches about women's weight, the old paths lead only to dead ends. We must boldly strike out in new directions.

CHAPTER 3

Find Out Why You're Overweight

Obesity is not a single disease, but a variety of conditions.

—*C. Wayne Callaway, M.D.*
George Washington University

Under the old ways of thinking about weight, you'd now be asked to consider how many calories you consume and how little you exercise. In Part 3, we'll explore the multiple ways to be fat in detail. But for a preliminary self-diagnosis right now, simply dig out a pen or pencil and jot "Y" for yes or "N" for no beside the following statements. Under the new paradigm of weight control, *these* are the kinds of questions you need to ask:

N 1. Do the men in your family get bald in their thirties or even their twenties?

Y 2. Do you frequently feel cold when others are warm?

N 3. Do you often have the feeling that everything is unreal?

N 4. When you try on a dress that fits just right on the top, is it too tight on the bottom?

Y 5. Do you often have great willpower for days, then suddenly pig out and blow your whole diet?

Y 6. Do you have a credit card bill you can't afford to pay?

N 7. Was either of your parents an alcoholic or addicted to drugs?

Y 8. Did you start gaining weight after being fired, the death of a child, or some other loss?

Y 9. Do you consume more than half of your daily calories after 6 P.M.?

N 10. Do you often or sometimes have the feeling that your body is not really yours?

N 11. Do you have any "wispy-haired" sisters?

Y 12. Do you sometimes feel out of control, stuff yourself with food, then later feel guilty about it?

Y 13. Do you often feel stressed just while going about your normal daily routine?

Y 14. Do you feel unsupported by the people closest to you?

N 15. Do you sometimes feel as if you're made up of two (or more) people, as if your mind is "split up"?

N 16. Do you have dry, scaly skin, a puffy face and eyes, or dry, brittle nails and hair?

Y 17. Do you have certain "forbidden foods" you sometimes eat uncontrollably?

Y 18. Do you often feel guilty?

N 19. When someone has an ignorant opinion or wastes your time, do you tell them about it so they'll shape up?

N 20. Did you begin gaining weight shortly after you started taking a medication?

Y 21. Do you have home repairs (a damaged roof or gutters, for example) that you never have the time or money to fix?

N 22. Do you feel foggy or have trouble concentrating and remembering things?

N 23. Can you remember some events in your past so vividly you have the feeling you're reliving them?

N 24. Do you have white skin spots or prematurely gray hair (one gray hair before the age of thirty)?

Y 25. Do some of those horrible stories about injustice on the nightly news make you just want to lash out?

Y 26. If your child gets sick, does day care suddenly become a crisis?

N 27. Do you find it impossible to sleep because the new baby keeps crying?

Y 28. Do you sometimes feel as if someone else inside your body is deciding what to do, almost as if your body has a mind of its own?

Y 29. Is your waist suddenly getting thicker as you grow older?

N 30. Are your cholesterol, blood sugar, blood pressure, and triglycerides all normal?

Y 31. Do you find it very hard to resist bad habits?
X 32. Are you taking pills for depression or high blood pressure?
N 33. Do you have velvety patches of skin on the back of your
        neck?
N 34. Is your sore back becoming a regular backache?
N 35. Did you gain weight after you quit smoking?
Y 36. Do you have two or more children?
N 37. Do you struggle with unwanted body hair, particularly on
        your arms, tummy, chin, or upper lip?
Y 38. Did you start dieting before you were eighteen?
N 39. When you walk, are you sometimes or often aware of each
        step you take?
N 40. Do you starve yourself all day and then eat ravenously at
        dinner?
Y 41. Do you tend to gain weight in the winter and lose it in the
        summer?
Y 42. Is it hard for you to get your work done on time because
        the phone keeps ringing?
Y 43. Are you frequently exhausted and depressed, although
        everything in your life is just fine?
N 44. Do you wake up several times a night for a snack, then have
        no appetite for breakfast?
Y 45. When people annoy you, do you harbor a silent grudge
        until you can no longer stand it, then suddenly explode?
N 46. Have you been gaining about a pound a year since your
        twenties?
N 47. Have you ever lost or gained five pounds or more in a sin-
        gle week?
Y 48. When you cheat on your diet, do you tell yourself, "I'm so
        stupid. Now I've blown my whole diet. I'll never lose
        weight."
N 49. Have you been trying to have a baby without success?
Y 50. Do you believe most people would cheat on their taxes if
        they thought they could get away with it?

Look back over the questions to which you answered yes and
write the numbers here: _____ 19 _____.
Now match your answers with the multiple ways to be fat below.
The estimates in parentheses are best guesses drawn from the med-

ical literature. The numbers add up to more than 100 percent because many women have "nesting syndromes" (two or more syndromes together). Just knowing these ways to be fat exist can help you understand those fat "spurts" in your own life with new insight.

1. HEALTHY FAT

(May affect nearly half of women currently on diets.) If you answered yes to questions 4, 29, 30, 35, and 46, here's a big surprise. Your fat may be healthy! We're often told that even a few extra pounds will damage our health but, in fact, as we'll discuss more fully in Chapter 5, this has never been proved. One woman with healthy fat put it this way: "I'm *not* depressed or angry. I don't binge when I'm stressed. I've never dieted much, I don't take medications, and I'm not even tired. My life is going quite well. I seldom get discouraged. In fact, I'm happy, healthy, self-confident, and usually have tons of energy. I exercise regularly. I'm just *fat*." If she sounds a lot like you, you'll want to pay special attention to Chapter 7, "Do You Have Healthy Fat?"

2. DAILY HASSLES FAT

(Probably affects up to 80 percent of women with unhealthy fat to some extent.) If you answered yes to questions 6, 13, 21, 26, 34, and 42, this surprisingly common way to be fat may be your problem. It's easy to notice the big stresses in our lives (loss of a job, moving cross-country, getting a divorce). But it's those little hassles like being stuck in traffic, rushing to finish too many chores in too little time, misplacing our checkbooks, or nursing a sick family member that often make our waistlines expand. Fat is especially likely to pile on during times of added responsibility when we're afraid we can't handle the challenge—maybe even if we don't consume extra calories. Although some women lose weight in response to stress, many others report gaining a bundle of weight while going to graduate school or after being promoted to a better-paying but more pressured job. Why? Low confidence in response to stress may play a big role. When Janet D. Allan at the University of Texas Health Science Center in San Antonio asked women why they gained weight, 80 percent of white women, 65 percent of black women, and 42.5 percent of Mexican-American women cited "life stress" as a major culprit. So perhaps this is why Melissa, the coed I bet five bucks on in college, lost her weight challenge to Becca: she was flunking out of school that spring and, in fact, didn't return the following fall.

3. DEPRESSION FAT

(Affects 10 to 20 percent of overweight women.) A yes to questions 8, 18, 41, and 48 indicates you may have gained weight because you're depressed. The Germans call this unhealthy type of fat *Kummerspeck*, which means "fat of sorrow." The word was coined shortly after World War I to describe the weight women put on after their loved ones had gone off to war or been killed, weight gains that could not be explained by calories alone. This type of weight gain frequently occurs in a spurt, often after a deep personal loss. One contemporary example: shortly after her father died at age fifty-two from a heart attack, actress Marilu Henner reported gaining 25 pounds in just seven weeks.

One especially telling study linking depression with rapid weight gain was done on fifty-five women who'd just been imprisoned. As they went to jail, those women most worried about separating from their children and families and losing control of their lives were the most likely to become depressed over the next six months. They were also the most likely to gain unhealthy fat. Winter Fat, which you may have if you answered yes to question 41, appears to be a subtype of this condition.

4. LAZY THYROID FAT

(Affects about 10 percent of overweight women.) If you answered yes to questions 2, 16, 22, 24, and 43, this could be your problem. At first glance, this condition, called *hypothyroidism*, looks like a purely physiological problem, because the thyroid gland is not working properly. This way to be fat can also be treated with medication, which adds to the notion that it's "only" a physical disease. Many women struggling with Lazy Thyroid Fat, however, say their thyroids went haywire only after a particularly stressful period in their lives—and doctors are also finding stress plays a bigger role in triggering thyroid problems than was previously thought.

Ridha Arem, M.D., an endocrinologist at Baylor College of Medicine in Houston, notes that stress isn't the only trigger for thyroid problems—but it's an important one. "The biochemical cascade that links the brain to the immune system is at the root of how mental stress triggers thyroid imbalance," he writes in *The Thyroid Solution*. Women struggling with Depression Fat and Post-Trauma Fat frequently also have lazy thyroids.

5. ANGER FAT
(May affect 20 percent of women with unhealthy fat.) If you answered yes to questions 14, 19, 25, 45, and 50, this may be your problem. It's also a particularly dangerous way to be fat. Hostile anger (often a sign of extreme stress) goes hand in hand in both men and women with more unhealthy fat and other risk factors for chronic disease, including high blood pressure, high blood sugar, high insulin levels, and poor cholesterol profiles. In the Healthy Women Study, conducted jointly by researchers at the University of Helsinki and the University of Pittsburgh, middle-aged women who frequently felt intensely angry and openly expressed their anger at other people gained more unhealthy fat over a thirteen-year period than less hostile women. They also gained more weight overall and had higher insulin levels.

Duke University psychiatrist Redford Williams estimates that 20 percent of people in the United States are carrying around enough anger for it to be hazardous to their hearts. But Anger Fat isn't just a U.S. ill. In Great Britain, a University of London survey of more than ten thousand civil servants revealed a clear link between poorly paid work, anger, and excess weight: those lowest in the pecking order in the worst-paying jobs were the angriest—and the fattest.

6. AND 7. THE TWO BINGE-EATING SYNDROMES
(Affects about 10 percent of overweight women, plus millions of women who aren't fat.) Did you answer yes to questions 5, 12, 17, and 31? Then you may have a full-fledged Binge-Eating Disorder (BED). Definitely stress-triggered, BED often goes hand in hand with depression, anxiety, self-consciousness, body-image problems, loneliness, and possibly Post-Trauma Fat. About 30 percent of women who show up in weight-loss clinics and 10 to 15 percent of women who try commercial programs like Weight Watchers or Jenny Craig struggle with this condition. Once they start eating,

they feel so compulsive they often can't stop. Binge eaters often feel warmer than other people and tend to sweat a lot (the result of their bodies working overtime to metabolize and store all that food). Other signs of this common syndrome include: chaotic eating, overeating during both meals and binges, and feeling panicky and out of control. Tending to gain and lose weight in spurts, a binge eater is more likely than other overweight women to have regular weight fluctuations exceeding 20 pounds (a major risk for heart disease).

A variation of binge eating is the Binge-Starve Syndrome, or what might be called "diet-induced fat." Are you ready for this one? It's caused by eating *too little*. If you answered yes to questions 38, 40, and 47, this may be your problem. In some women, this way to be fat may even be triggered by dieting. In one study conducted at Yale University, 45 percent of binge eaters reported that dieting preceded their first binge, whereas 55 percent said bingeing preceded their first diet. The 27 percent of adolescent girls in the United States who say they're at the right weight but are nonetheless dieting to get thinner are at high risk for this disorder.

8. POLYCYSTIC OVARY SYNDROME (PCOS)

(Affects 8 to 10 percent of overweight women, up to 20 percent of those severely overweight.) If you answered yes to questions 1, 11, 33, 37, and/or 49, you may have this surprisingly common hormonal imbalance. Far from being rare, this hormonal disorder afflicts up to 20 percent of severely overweight women. In a 1991 issue of the *Journal of Endocrinology*, University of London endocrinologist Stephen Franks even titles his review on the subject "The Ubiquitous Polycystic Ovary." A study published in the *American Journal of Medicine* calls PCOS "the most common endocrine disorder in women of reproductive age." At least half, and perhaps as many as 80 percent, of women with PCOS are overweight. Many are also infertile. Yet this "ubiquitous" way to be fat is almost never diagnosed, and very few women know they have it. Even most doctors don't know about PCOS. When University of Pittsburgh epidemiologist Evelyn Talbott did a study on PCOS in a journal put out by the American Heart Association, she observed she, too, was "surprised" the syndrome is so common.

One of the most obvious signs of PCOS, other than extra weight, is thick, coarse body hair on a woman's arms and face, particularly those in areas where men grow sideburns, beards, or mustaches. Many women with this type of fat have acne, husky voices, and broad shoulders. This is one way to be fat that definitely *won't* go away just by exercising more and eating less. First, the hormonal imbalance has to be treated.

9. NIGHT-EATING SYNDROME

(Affects about 10 percent of overweight women.) Do you start out in the morning with no appetite for breakfast, then grow increasingly depressed as the day wears on, until by nightfall you're ravenous? If so, and if you also answered yes to questions 9 and 44, you may be struggling with Night-Eating Syndrome. First described in 1955 by Albert Stunkard at the University of Pennsylvania, Night-Eating Syndrome (NES) has been found in up to 27 percent of seriously overweight people, and about 10 percent of those who go to obesity clinics. In one clinic study, a whopping 64 percent of extremely overweight women had this disorder. In another study, so did 75 percent of female recovering alcoholics who identified themselves as binge eaters. Women who are fat in this way report the problem escalates when they're under stress. Night eaters have higher-than-normal cortisol levels around the clock. Between midnight and 4 A.M., they also have extremely low levels of melatonin, a hormone that induces sleep and resets the body's biological clock.

10. POST-PREGNANCY FAT

(Affects all new mothers to some extent, some far more seriously than others.) It doesn't take a rocket scientist to know that pregnancy triggers weight gain in most women. If you answered yes to questions 27 and 36, you may be struggling with Post-Pregnancy Fat. We're often told we should be able to have two or three kids without gaining more than three or four pounds. That's highly misleading and may cause enormous frustration and body-image problems among women who believe it. Pregnancy changes your hormones in many complex ways that can cause you to retain weight after the birth of a child, even if you don't consume extra calories. Generally, the women most likely to stay fat after childbirth are those who gained the most while they were pregnant. Other factors that can play into how much weight you'll retain after a pregnancy and how hard you'll struggle to lose it include:

- your age (women in their twenties tend to lose maternity fat faster and more easily than those in their thirties and forties, but teen moms may gain more and have a harder time taking it off)
- your race (black moms are twice as likely as white moms to retain 20 or more pounds after childbirth)
- your height (short women are often encouraged to gain as much as tall women, but they may wind up fatter as a result)
- smoking status (45 percent of women who quit smoking when they became pregnant gained 10 pounds or more as a result of the pregnancy and quitting combined. But it's still best to stop smoking!)
- your genes (if your mother put on weight when she had kids, you may follow suit)
- your financial situation (poor mothers are six times more likely to be obese than rich mothers)

Is Post-Pregnancy Fat healthy? Some of it can be (if it's in the hips and thighs); but after pregnancy, many women also accumulate more fat in their visceral cells. We'll talk a lot more about this in Chapter 16.

11. MEDICATION-CAUSED FAT

(Affects up to 90 percent of women on some medications.) Did your diet plateau or did you gain weight after you started a new medication? Dozens of prescription and over-the-counter drugs can cause weight gain in certain women. Some drugs slow down your metabolism. Others cause cravings for sweets. Still others promote fat storage. Among the worst offenders are the tricyclic antidepressants like amitriptyline (which causes weight gain in as many as 89 percent of women who take it). Since more than 51 million prescriptions for tricyclics are written each year in the United States alone, millions of women undoubtedly have Medication-Caused Fat and don't know it. If you answered yes to questions 20 or 32, you may be one of them. We'll give a detailed list of the many drugs that can make you fat in Chapter 17.

12. Post-Trauma Fat

(Affects as many as 25 percent of chronically overweight women.) Even as many as thirty to sixty years after childhood sexual abuse, many women are still eating to assuage their pain—and struggling with Post-Trauma Fat. If you answered yes to questions 3, 7, 10, 15, 23, 28, and 39, you may be one of them. At any sign of threat, these women's bodies becomes hypervigilant and flooded with cortisol, a hormone that promotes fat storage. Stress for women with Post-Trauma Fat differs from ordinary stress in that any situation that resembles the previous trauma can stir up deep-seated fears and lead to overeating. Women who've collected Post-Trauma Fat may be easily startled and show exaggerated stress responses to the smallest surprises (a stranger's asking for directions, for example). They may also suffer flashbacks or "numb out." In such an unpredictable emotional milieu, even the most outwardly confident woman may frequently feel inwardly shaken. In one weight clinic in San Diego, 60 percent of female patients who'd been sexually molested or raped as little girls were at least 50 pounds overweight—and 35 percent were 50 to 100 pounds too heavy. What's more, they couldn't seem to lose weight, no matter how hard they tried. In a Texas A&M study of women with eating disorders, 52 percent had symptoms of post-traumatic stress disorder (PTSD). Past sexual abuse is also sometimes associated with Binge-Eating Syndrome.

Fortunately, the human brain and body are blessed with amazing resilience. Rachel Yehuda at Mount Sinai Hospital in New York City has found that of Holocaust victims who once had PTSDs, one-fourth had recovered and no longer suffered symptoms. They also no longer had elevated stress hormones. Understanding this condition is the first step toward regaining control.

The Nesting Syndromes:
Combinations of Ways to Be Fat

If more than one of these ways to be fat rings a bell, you may be fat in more than one way. Like many women, you may have what I call nesting syndromes. Samantha, a New York City publicity manager, is a prime example. She currently weighs 193 pounds, having gained about 50 of them in the past year. Two years ago, she considered herself "happily married" with one baby girl and was trying to get pregnant again when her divorce-attorney husband came home late one Friday and announced he'd fallen in love with a client. Over the next year during her messy divorce, Samantha went into an emotional and physical tailspin. Her periods became "inexplicably" heavy, and she began focusing all her anxiety on her heavy bleeding. On her doctor's advice, she had a hysterectomy (one way to be fat). After the surgery, she became deeply depressed about never having another baby (a form of Depression Fat), so her doctor in his wisdom prescribed a weight-causing antidepressant. Now she had Medication-Caused Fat, too! Samantha soon became obsessive-compulsive. Some days she couldn't leave her apartment until she'd checked the front door three or four times to make sure it was locked. To counteract this new "symptom" (really a side effect of the first medication), her doctor prescribed yet another drug. By now, Samantha's weight was careening out of control. All the beautiful clothes in her closet no longer fit. The stress from a promotion to more responsibility at work only made matters worse. At her last checkup, her blood pressure had soared. (Let's hope her doctor doesn't prescribe a blood pressure drug next!) Sam diets for days and then binges (especially on Friday nights about the time her ex came home with his news). She tries to exercise, but working out frequently seems like just one more impossible chore. She's currently on three drugs (counting Premarin), any one of which could be slowing down her metabolism. Clearly, Samantha's life has spiraled out of control. To get out of this morass, she needs a little help from the weight-control winners who understand how she feels. Fortunately, that's just who we're now going to meet.

CHAPTER 4

Superconfidence and How to Get It

Life is not easy for any of us. But what of that? We must have perseverance and above all confidence in ourselves.

—Madame Curie

When we're struggling with our weight, we often tell ourselves, "Once I get thin, I'm really going to get my act together." Winners report they often got their acts together *before* they kept the weight off. These are the kinds of decisions some winners had to make in their lives before they could finally take charge:

- "I had to get up my nerve to start looking for a better job."—Denise, thirty-two, who had Daily Hassles Fat
- "I had to find a doctor who would tell me what was wrong with me and fix my hormonal imbalance."—Carrie, thirty-five, who had PCOS
- "I had to dump my abusive boyfriend and talk about being raped."—Vicky, fifty-nine, who had Post-Trauma Fat
- "I had to realize I'm healthy at 182 pounds. I exercise regularly, I eat right, and my body is beautiful."—Lynn, thirty-four, who had Healthy Fat
- "I had to stop taking antidepressants and start asking who God meant for me to be and what he wants me to do."—Arlene, forty, who had Medication-Caused Fat
- "I had to get outside more, enjoy the sunshine, and reset my biological clock."—Beth, thirty-two, who had a combination of Winter Fat and Night-Eating Syndrome

The list goes on and on, as individual and varied as the women who win. Superconfidence isn't superhuman. It unfolds naturally when how we're feeling and what we're thinking are in harmony with the choices we're making and how we're living our lives.

Winners prize their individuality and find unique solutions to the challenges of managing their weight. It's almost as if someone had already told them there are multiple ways of being fat, as if they had resolved, "All right, then there must be multiple ways to get thin." They ask questions until they understand all their options. Then they build on their own strengths. They become what University of Massachusetts stress researcher Jon Kabat-Zinn calls "the scientists of their own bodies." But they go even beyond that. They become the scientists of their own lives. They ask astute questions, make their own "best guesses" about the right course of action, experiment to test their theories, and trust their own observations. In the end, they develop individualized strategies that *they* alone decide will work best for them. As one superconfident woman who beat Night-Eating Syndrome put it, "I continually studied my body and my eating patterns much as if I were a bug under a microscope. I became very curious about me."

Sarah, forty-four, a jewelry designer and self-described "caffeine-holic" who once drank as many as twelve cups of coffee and a liter of diet Coke every day, insists she finally lost 15 pounds of Daily Hassles Fat mostly by switching to herbal tea. "I know it sounds crazy because there are no calories in coffee and diet Coke," she says. "But it worked." The current research suggests Sarah's solution may not have been so crazy. By going cold turkey on caffeine, she probably reduced her stress. And it's stress (not just calories) that matters most in many of the multiple ways to be fat.

In her constant search for answers, Sarah followed the weight-control winners' axiom: experiment until you find something that works. Then do more of it.

Weight-control winners do that a lot. Pam Grout, a freelance journalist in Kansas, claims she dropped 10 pounds in three weeks just by taking thirty deep breaths every day. As the single mom of a one-year-old at the time, she recalls in her book *Jumpstart Your Metabolism*, "I had about as much energy as a dead goldfish." When an infomercial promised she could become more energetic with deep breathing, she reasoned that since she was *already* breathing, it shouldn't be "too much trouble to breathe a little more." So she started taking ten deep breaths three times a day. That's when she lost the 10 pounds. Under the old calories in, calories out, paradigm, this woman's experience sounds ludicrous and should never have worked. But it did. And when you think about it, you realize there was something authentic about her "off-the-wall" solution. The technique she hit on wasn't all that far removed from the stress-reducing "relaxation response" devised by Harvard's Herbert Benson and now used in university-based weight-control programs.

Playful and curious, winners rise above their problems, often with a sense of humor. They're able to laugh at their foibles. On her way home from a particularly harrowing day at the office, Heather, who had Binge-Eating Fat, told herself, "Boy, when I get home tonight, I'm going to eat everything in the refrigerator. I'm going to eat a whole gallon of ice cream, a dozen eggs, six Sara Lee cakes, twelve TV dinners, and a gallon of milk. I may even eat the refrigerator door." The more she exaggerated her fears of bingeing, the more she laughed at herself. Once she got home, she made a bee-line for the refrigerator, acting silly and shouting, "Here I come, Fridge, I'm going to destroy you! I'm going to eat you all up." Guess what? To her great surprise, she wasn't hungry! Laughing, she headed upstairs for a warm, relaxing bath and was later able to satisfy her hunger with a small salad and a cup of soup.

Why did *that* work? Well, it may have worked partly because she inadvertently hit on a powerful psychological tool called "paradoxical intention," devised by psychoanalyst Viktor E. Frankl. Heather used what Frankl called "the specifically human capacity" to detach herself from her fears with humor—and thereby lessen the distress that usually led to a binge.

Laughing at yourself as a way to transcend problems has been known to people for eons. But since paradoxical intention as a scientific principle is a bit tricky to understand, let's look at another example. This one doesn't involve weight loss, but it comes from Frankl and clearly illustrates the technique. A young physician was so afraid of perspiring in public that he sought therapy. The problem was that his private anxieties brought on the very public perspiration he feared. Frankl advised him that if the situation recurred and he found himself perspiring, he should deliberately show people how much he could sweat. Over the next week, whenever the young doctor met anyone who triggered his anxiety, he told himself, "I only sweated out a quart before, but now I'm going to pour out at least ten quarts!" He literally *strained* to sweat. As a result, within a week he was able to rid himself permanently of a phobia he'd had for four years. Fear causes what we're afraid of (in this young doctor's case, sweating; in Heather's case, a binge). If one strains to do precisely what one fears most, Frankl noted, "the wind is taken out of the sails of anxiety." Distress disappears.

The Winners' Way: Self-Efficacy

Such solutions—taking ten deep breaths three times a day or making a joke of eating the refrigerator door—were not just "accidental discoveries." The women thought of them because they did not let the situation get out of hand and become bigger than they were. They stayed on top of their problems and kept looking for solutions. Any idea that came to mind, even if it was silly, they tried. When a strategy worked, they did more of it. When it didn't work, they tried something else.

When we're struggling with our weight, we feel out of control. Anxious to get back in control, we tend to look for only the most "authoritative" solutions. We run to doctors, weight-control clinics, exercise trainers, nutritionists, and other diet gurus, failing to notice that the only real solution to our problems lies within us. Only *we* can become the authors of our own lives.

Women in our culture are often taught to trust others to improve their health. But it's how much a woman learns to trust *herself* and her own answers that determines whether she'll take charge of her weight for life. Since the late 1970s, hundreds of medical studies have shown that self-confidence—or what Stanford University psychologist Albert Bandura calls strong *self-efficacy*—is more important, in the long run, than any mechanical prescription, be it a pill, diet, exercise routine, or medical procedure.

Women with "high perceived self-efficacy" (in other words, those who strongly *believe* they can succeed) are more able to achieve whatever they set out to do. They're more able to quit smoking, beat alcoholism, reduce chronic pain, recover from a heart attack, interrupt panic attacks, and even stay mentally sharp into old age. Strong self-confidence helps diabetics control their blood sugar better and helps heart-disease patients keep their cholesterol down. Strong faith in themselves and their own inner radar also helps weight-control winners determine why they're overweight, lose unhealthy fat, bounce back when the going gets tough, and keep the weight off.

Just calmly *believing* you can lose weight may work even better than diet pills. In one classic study, Catherine A. Chambliss and E. J. Murray gave overweight women sugar pills but described the pills as medications that would help them gain self-control. Once women lost weight, the pills were discontinued. Women who believed the pills had done all the work quickly regained their lost weight. Those told the truth—that the pills were merely sugar and they'd really succeeded on their own efforts—continued to lose. Ordinary, frustrated women had become weight-loss winners simply by learning to believe in themselves.

Acquiring the self-confidence to lose weight your way can also help you *maintain* your losses. Albert J. Stunkard and his coworkers at the University of Pennsylvania divided overweight women into three groups: one group got diet pills, the second group got pills plus lessons in self-management, the third group got only self-management lessons. Once the treatments stopped, women in the first two groups who'd taken the pills regained most of the weight they'd lost. Why? Because they believed in the pills, not in themselves. Women in the third group, who had acquired the self-trust to lose weight without magic bullets, still maintained their losses a year later.

The healing power of belief may help explain why some women lose weight on the wackiest diets. It's not the diet. It's their *belief* in the diet. It's the "doctor within" that really makes the fat go away. Once these same women go off the diet or no longer trust that it will work for them, they regain all their lost weight. Binge eaters are extremely responsive to the superconfidence effect. In one study, binge eaters reduced their binge frequency by 72 percent just by taking sugar pills. If some kook would come out with a book called *The Anti-Binge Diet* filled with a bunch of weird food combinations (don't eat green beans with cabbage, for example), you can darned well bet TV talk-show stages would soon be crowded with former binge eaters honestly swearing it was the miracle diet that saved their lives. Are women stupid for believing such nonsense? No. They're just unaware of their own power. Superconfidence is the power that activates the healer within.

We tend to notice a dynamo in the office and think, "Now *there's* a confident woman." But confidence in one's ability to succeed isn't a global strength. You can be calmly confident inside when it's time to surf the Internet, sell real estate, or give a speech but have no confidence at all in your abilities to sing opera, pilot a plane, or lose fat for life. Self-efficacy is built on *acquired skills*. It doesn't just bubble up spontaneously out of your personality.

Marcella, a travel agent I know, is a whiz at organizing. She employs about thirty people and grosses about $20 million a year. She can hop on a plane at a moment's notice, zip halfway around the world, and arrive in Hong Kong, looking as freshly rested as if she slept all night at the Hilton. Her Long Island home is superbly self-decorated and her flower gardens are among the most charming I've ever seen. In many areas of her life—from making money and traveling to decorating with flair—her self-efficacy is so high it's off the charts. But when it comes to controlling her weight, she confesses that for the past five years, she hasn't even tried to slim down. Five feet tall and 153 pounds (give or take a few), she simply gave up. Though confident in a thousand other ways, she has no weight-control self-efficacy at all.

Self-efficacy may sound a lot like self-love, but the two concepts are quite different. Loving yourself (important as that is) doesn't automatically lead to gaining the resources you need to slim down. You can love yourself, even adore yourself, and stay fat. (Many women, in fact, do.) Or you can adore yourself and also acquire the knowledge and skills to slim down. Self-efficacy involves how *capable* you feel about achieving your healthiest weight. Self-love has to do with whether you feel you *deserve* to be thin, an entirely different matter.

Self-efficacy may also sound a lot like old-fashioned motivation or willpower. But it isn't that, either. Just being motivated to lose weight doesn't mean you'll acquire the facts and understanding you need to succeed. If you follow the wrong prescriptions for your individual way to be fat, you'll never get thin, no matter how "motivated" you may be.

Strong self-efficacy or superconfidence is an ever-adapting, ever-changing skill that's ready-made, almost biologically designed, to match your constantly adapting, ever-changing mind and body. Rules invented by anyone but you will fail when the going gets tough. When you're tired at the end of a long day or you just lost your job, lectures from your doctor, a nutritionist, or even the Queen of England won't keep you from eating that doughnut. Yet no matter how subtly your body's chemistry changes, how much your moods rise and fall, whether you've had a good day or a bad one, your superconfidence is there on the job, ready to take charge.

So how do you learn this essential skill?

Weight-control winners calmly step back and observe where their eating self-efficacy is weak and then strengthen their skills in those areas. One woman with Binge-Eating Syndrome, for example, had strong confidence in her ability to resist food when she was reading but none at all when she was watching TV. (Her solution: she gave her TV set to the Salvation Army.) Monica, a thirty-nine-year-old Philadelphia nurse with Night-Eating Syndrome, could resist overeating when she was angry, anxious, or depressed during the day but had no self-trust around food when she was home alone at night. Part of her solution required getting out of the house in the evenings by joining a bowling team and a community theater group. A third woman with Anger Fat needed to learn how to handle her rage without exploding (she eventually forgave her ex-husband), whereas a winner with Depression Fat had to work through her grief over her father's suicide and move on with her life.

So here we have a multiplicity of solutions to a multiplicity of problems. One woman lost weight partly by giving away her TV. Another joined a bowling team and a theater group. A third forgave her ex-husband. A fourth worked through the grief caused by her father's suicide. The ways to get thin, like the ways to be fat, are diverse and not always readily apparent in the busy complexity of our lives. None of these winners consciously knew about the multiple ways to be fat. They had never heard about Binge-Eating Syndrome, Depression Fat, Post-Trauma Fat, or the other syndromes now emerging. They found their solutions through trial and learning, and it took many of them years to win. They were true pioneers. If they'd known what you're about to learn, they could have taken shortcuts and found their answers much sooner, the way you're about to do.

The Biology of Superconfidence

Years ago, *Saturday Review of Literature* editor Norman Cousins wrote about the "biology of hope." Dr. Herbert Benson of Harvard Medical School has written about the "biology of belief." In his books and on a popular PBS series, northern California cardiologist Dean Ornish has documented the "biology of intimacy." Now Dr. Albert Bandura has shown there's also a "biology of self-confidence."

This biology, as it turns out, is exactly the same biology that releases fat-dissolving effort hormones (called catecholamines) while at the same time shutting down the most important hormone involved in unhealthy fat storage (the distress hormone cortisol). In other words, superconfidence keeps your body mobilizing fat without storing it in your unhealthiest fat cells. In the next few chapters, you'll see how superconfidence can change your biology right down to the level of the fat cell in a way that helps you lose weight and keep it off.

Bandura first began observing how self-confidence changes your biology, particularly your stress hormones, when he studied people with snake and spider phobias. One study involved people so terrified of spiders that some had given up gardening or refused to sit in the yard. Just the thought of seeing a spider made their effort hormones (the fat-burning catecholamines) soar. Once they became so terrified they no longer even tried to cope with a situation involving spiders, their effort hormones took a nosedive and their distress or defeat hormone cortisol kicked in. Yet when these same people learned to master their fears by learning how to handle spiders safely, they could confidently let spiders crawl on their arms while all their stress hormones remained under control and their bodies stayed calm.

Catecholamines are the only hormones in the human body that play any serious role in breaking down fat. What's more, catecholamine secretions, Bandura explains, "essentially mirror" the strength of your beliefs in your ability to handle a challenge. Catecholamines and confidence are like two people on a seesaw. When your confidence is superhigh, catecholamine levels are normal and fat burn-

ing is just perking along. When your confidence is low, catecholamine secretions rise to the point that you feel so helpless you give
up in defeat. That's when fat release stops and cortisol kicks in, storing fat deep in your abdomen. It's catecholamines coupled with cortisol that give you that spare tire.

Strong self-confidence interrupts this cycle. Just *believing* you
can cope with your problems takes away feelings of threat. Situations that once triggered high-cortisol reactions—such as being
angry at a coworker or feeling lonely and depressed on a Saturday
night—can be managed without physiological stress when you
strengthen your ability to handle the situation. This helps explain
why women with high confidence are also most likely to win their
weight-control battles.

Fortunately, the kind of confidence these women display is not
the kind that comes from being perfect, beautiful, popular, and
beloved from the start. Superconfidence isn't some illusive magic
wand. It's a craft you can *learn*, built step-by-step on acquired skills.

Think of something—anything—you do especially well. Maybe
it's your job. Maybe you're a good cook, a wonderful storyteller, or
a fine gardener. Maybe you knit lovely afghans, arrange flowers
with flair, have a special way with animals, or organize rummage
sales better than anyone else. Now consider how you built your
mastery and confidence in this area. This "talent" didn't come to
you out of the blue. It developed because you learned some secrets
about what you do well that other people haven't bothered to learn.
Over time, by paying attention to what worked, you gained special
insights. In this area of your life, you gained the craft of confidence.

The same principle applies to gaining confidence about your
eating behavior. You don't need to acquire some nebulous "willpower" or whip yourself up into some superpsychological state to
take charge of your weight for life. You simply need to gain a few
simple skills, so you can address your individual way to be fat.
There are multiple ways to be fat, but you don't have to solve them
all. That's where you have a huge advantage over the doctors:
they're supposed to cure everybody who walks into their office.
Since there are so many ways to be fat, that gets pretty tricky. You,
on the other hand, need to solve only one problem (or, more likely,
one *set* of problems): your own. That's why when it comes to weight
loss, you have a big advantage over even the world's best experts:

you know your own body. Nobody knows your body better than you do. It's like your own little laboratory.

Resourceful winners report that distress around food lessens once they learn how to handle "threatening" situations more calmly. Francine, fifty-two, a Miami yoga instructor and highly observant scientist of her own body who recovered from a heart-hazardous case of Anger Fat, reports:

> For years, whenever my stepmother would call, I would not even *feel* the verbal barbs she hurled at me. I'd just passively and numbly take them all in. Then I'd get off the phone and inhale a quart of ice cream. Slowly, I came to recognize the pain she was inflicting. I also realized she'd never change. She'd always be a very weak, insecure, troubled woman—her own worst enemy, really. After that, whenever she called, I made a relaxed, conscious effort to observe her vicious criticism but not respond to it. I kept my mind and body aware and alert yet centered and still, so afterward I wasn't at all distressed and felt no need to eat. Once I realized I could control my own responses and stay in that pool of calmness where she could no longer hurt me, 75 pounds just melted away.

Many people would say Francine should have vented her anger, asserted herself, and told her stepmother to go straight to hell. But such advice might only have led to more Anger Fat. By becoming the scientist of her own body and solving her problem *her* way, Francine found a healing solution that worked. As a result, she reports also acquiring a deep inner peace.

We're often taught that being superconfident means you always need to stay in charge of *others*, that a confident woman has a "commanding presence" and displays her power simply by how boldly she can strut through a room, or speak at a conference, or bark orders at other people, bending them to her will. Given high-wattage super-achievers as role models, we're taught superconfidence is displayed in powerful *action*. But as Francine's story illustrates, superconfidence is more an inner mental attitude than an outwardly visible action or behavior. Real superconfidence springs from a learned ability to keep your mind/body calm, relaxed, and at peace, so you don't feel out of control. Many materially powerful women are secretly nervous wrecks inside. We're talking here about a power much greater than status, wealth, or worldly accomplishments. We're talking about the power to control one's own emotions and attain a deep inner peace. Superconfidence is an inside job.

Since superconfidence is built on skills much as you'd master a craft, how do you develop it? The insights gleaned from weight-control winners suggest that this robust self-confidence is both deepened and broadened in four principal ways:

1. finding out why you're fat (by embracing your uniqueness)
2. talking or listening to others like the winners who've already solved the same problem
3. being able to control your responses to stressful or taxing situations, so you feel less vulnerable and more in control
4. confidently facing your problems head-on

The first three skills will be completely explored in Part 3. But the fourth skill requires a bit more explanation right now. Many women who regain their lost weight tend to react to problems emotionally with anxiety, worry, depression, or anger. Winners, in contrast, calmly confront their problems head-on. They take direct action. In one provocative study at Kaiser Permanente in Oakland, California, most diet relapsers dealt with problems by trying to avoid or escape them. Overwhelmed by stress, they overate, smoked, drank alcohol, took tranquilizers, slept more, and wished their problems would go away. In contrast, 95 percent of weight-control winners in the same study faced their problems and began seeking solutions. They kept making an effort.

When they step on a scale and see they've gained 5 pounds, winners don't react emotionally with self-criticism ("Oh, my God, what will I do now? I've blown my whole diet. I'm a fool for eating that chocolate cake"). Such a reaction only blocks effort and increases stress. Instead, a winner sees those extra pounds merely as a problem she needs to make an extra effort to solve ("Okay, I've gained 5 pounds. I wonder if meditating thirty minutes a day this week and keeping a food diary will help?"). Winners also stay in effort-without-distress mode by exercising more than relapsers do and by turning to their friends or relatives in times of trouble for wise counsel and support. One winner who has kept 82 pounds off for three years reduced her distress levels by connecting and brainstorming regularly with a "diet buddy" on the Internet.

The Scientists of Their Own Bodies

Women struggling with their weight are such unique individuals it's impossible to make a single statement that applies to all. But if one melody runs through the stories of all winners, it's this: They reach what they alone determine to be their healthiest weights first, by finding out *why* they're fat, and, second, by searching until they find their own best answers. When they find a solution that works, they do more of it. When an idea doesn't work, they try something else. "I achieved my weight, my way" is the winners' constant refrain. There's a certain enthusiastic defiance in the way each woman boldly sings her own variation on this theme. One might even term "my weight, my way" the winner's battle cry—or, more aptly, her victory song.

Though winners are independently capable, they never operate in a vacuum. On the contrary, they stay completely open to all possibilities. They dig into medical journals, call doctors, join support groups, chat on the Internet, and pursue truth with a passion. They allow themselves to make mistakes without being critical or judgmental. When an experiment works, great. When it doesn't, no problem. They just try again—like the woman who designed twenty different diets for herself before she found one that worked. They seem to *collect* their mistakes and use them as tools to do better next time. The word *fail* isn't in their vocabulary.

Talking to weight-loss winners, I was reminded of Thomas Edison, who made most of his great discoveries through trial-and-error. When a coworker became discouraged during a particularly grueling series of experiments and insisted he'd "failed," Edison replied, "Shucks, we haven't failed. We now know a thousand things that won't work, so we're that much closer to finding what will." According to his son, Edison performed sixteen hundred experiments before he found the most suitable filament for a lightbulb and fifty thousand experiments to develop the accumulator battery. When told he was a "wizard," he would reply, "Pshaw. It's plain hard work that does it."

When Albert Einstein was stumped by a scientific problem, he would play the violin until a solution appeared. I found no weight-loss winners who played violins to find their answers. But I found many who prayed and meditated, several who wrote poetry or sang, and one who spent many precious hours sitting silently by herself on a pier under the stars, watching the moonlight glint off a lake as she sought answers. Losing weight is a science. But like all good science, it's also a creative act, calling for all the resourcefulness and self-expression needed for other forms of creativity.

Becoming the scientist of your own mind and body, of course, requires self-discipline. Yet, contrary to popular opinion, I'm convinced most overweight women already have strong self-discipline. During their lives, many overweight women have lost hundreds, even thousands of pounds. To find your weight, your way, you probably don't need to become *more* disciplined. You simply need to relax and direct your attention toward finding real solutions. You need to trust your intuition and the healer within. Intuition? But isn't that unscientific? Not for the great scientists, it's not. "It's too hard, and life is too short, to spend your time doing something because someone else has said it's important. You must feel the thing yourself," advised Isidor I. Rabi, a Nobel Prize–winning physicist. One of Einstein's favorite lines was: "This is so beautiful God could not have passed it up."

Denise, a thirty-two-year-old Los Angeles advertising copy-writer who struggled for years with Binge-Eating Syndrome but finally lost weight and has been at 121 pounds for three years, gives this rapid-fire advice to any woman who wants to find her own way: "Stay on your toes. Get on the Internet. Go to the library. Go here. Go there. Be alert. Think clearly. Take nothing for granted. Listen to your body. Stay open. *Connect.* Seek out other women struggling with similar problems. Brainstorm, ask questions, explore mutual answers. Do it your way, and be independent. But don't think you have to be all alone."

Of the many lessons winners teach, one of the wisest is this: the right answers are out there and also inside you—waiting. Answers for you as a unique individual. Answers that work. To find them, you just need a passion for knowing and a firm faith in your ability to dig out the truth.

PART TWO

Become the Scientist of Your Mind-Body

CHAPTER 5

Body Fat and Disease

A scientific truth [is] a hypothesis that might be adequate for the moment but [is] not to be preserved as an article of faith for all time.

—*Carl Jung*

In the whole history of medical science, the idea of viewing all fat as a disease is a recent development. In the second century, Galen, the brilliant Greek physician who wrote more than 125 medical books and whose work remained a medical standard for 1,300 years, identified two types of obesity: healthy (or "natural") and unhealthy (or "morbid"). Now, doctors on the cutting edge of weight-control research are once again returning to a view of fat much like that Galen proposed. Some fat is now viewed as healthy. Other fat is unhealthy and needs to be lost.

Weight-control winners knew it all the time. "The weight charts say I'm too heavy, but I don't care. I feel great at 165 pounds, and I'll never diet again," says Charlene, thirty-seven, an audiologist from a family of "big women" whose stout grandmother lived to ninety-three. Charlene has healthy fat. She eats nutritiously, bicycles daily, and has the energy of a bungee jumper. What about her blood pressure? "A little high," she replies defiantly. "So is my mother's. She's eighty-one, skis all winter, and has no signs of heart disease." After going on and off countless diets, Charlene finally decided to keep her fat.

You might think this was a fairly simple choice for her once she stopped spinning on the dieting merry-go-round long enough to think clearly. You might think that by choosing to stay heavy, she took the "easy" way out. Nothing could be further from the truth.

We have a myth in our culture that any woman who decides to stay heavy has somehow "copped out," that she's not emotionally or spiritually growing. But there is nothing stagnant about those winners who confidently decide to embrace their individuality. Respecting one's natural weight as being heavier than the popular ideas of what it means to be "sexy" requires great emotional, intellectual, and often even spiritual growth.

Many other winners, in contrast, had unhealthy fat and kept reinventing themselves until they found ways to lose it. So how did *they* succeed? Considering all the erroneous, misleading, or fraudulent information about weight in our culture, it wasn't easy. Most of them made many false starts and stops (some might erroneously call them "mistakes") before they hit on the truth. Some, like Charlene, tried to lose healthy fat many times before they confidently said, "Forget this. I'm going to find new ways to be healthy and heavy." Others with distressful, unhealthy fat mixed trial and learning with common sense, luck, and blind accident. Selena, who lives in Maine, created twenty different "diets" (really normal eating plans) before she finally invented one that would get her through the long winters without getting plump. Tammy, a manicurist in Houston, suddenly realized she had PCOS one day while doing a client's nails when the woman just happened to mention a neighbor who'd lost lots of weight after correcting a hormonal imbalance. A few winners took more than twenty years to find their own answers! They were true pioneers.

Fortunately, you needn't wait twenty years to learn what they discovered on their own initiative through trial and learning. Education is a shortcut to experience, and you can take that shortcut. Legitimate scientists often shake their heads in disbelief at all the crackpot diet advice in our society and wonder, "How can women be so stupid as to believe such nonsense?" Jules Hirsch of Rockefeller University has called the current anticarbohydrate craze a kind of "alchemy" in which "ignorance is turned into gold." But even the smartest and most confident women often become confused and misled by wrongheaded advice because we're never told how and why we gain fat. To find your own individual "winner's way" past all the misinformation about weight in our culture, it helps immensely to understand the nature and physiology of a fat cell. Any true path to fat loss must be grounded in physiology. Fat, after all, is a material substance; it doesn't magically evaporate into thin air. That's why the first shortcut to becoming a superconfident weight-control winner involves a short biology lesson.

Your Multiple Kinds of Fat Cells

The average woman's body contains about 25 to 35 billion fat cells. To envision that number, if you took 35 billion ordinary postage stamps and stretched them end to end, they would encircle the earth at the equator twenty-two times. If you were to weigh twice what you supposedly "should," according to those ideal weight charts, your body might contain as many as 100 to 125 billion fat cells. Most of us think of fat cells as a bunch of amorphous jellylike blobs that all look and act exactly alike. But, in fact, our bodies contain so many different kinds of fat cells scientists haven't even named them all yet. Just as there are multiple ways to be fat, there are multiple kinds of fat cells.

On the simplest level, fat comes in two colors: brown and white. Brown cells are designed to *burn* fat and keep the body warm. White cells are designed for fat *storage*.

Brown cells are common in hibernating animals. In humans, they're most active in babies. When you were a baby, your brown cells kept you toasty warm and could double your metabolic rate when you were exposed to a temperature no colder than 78 degrees. Now that you're an adult, your brown fat cells have atrophied and no longer burn fat. Still, some drug companies eye these dormant little brown-cell "furnaces" as prime candidates for a diet pill that would rev up our metabolism. If they could just find a way to switch our brown cells "back on," some researchers believe, they could jump-start our metabolism and cure all our fat woes. But so far, this idea hasn't panned out.

White fat cells are the kind you're trying to lose (or, more accurately, shrink) when you go on a diet. These white cells come in many different varieties, from small and compact to big and stretchy. They also vary dramatically, depending on their locations in the body. Thus, you have subcutaneous fat cells (under the skin), visceral fat cells (deep in the abdomen), femoral fat cells (in your thighs), gluteal fat cells (in your derriere), mammary fat cells (in

your breasts), and many other subtypes scientists are only beginning to classify. "Prefat" cells haven't become white fat cells yet. But
they're just waiting to turn into full-fledged white fat when all your
other cells are full. It's been said that if all our fat cells were full,
we'd each contain enough fat to stuff a small couch.

When you were a baby, many of your white fat cells were so
small they contained no fat. But as you grew bigger, your fat cells
got bigger. When you ran out of space in the fat cells you had, a
stress hormone called cortisol helped your prefat cells turn into
full-fledged fat cells, a process that can occur at any age. Even after
age sixty, your body will contain large numbers of prefat cells just
waiting to take on a little cream cheese or butter.

Once you add new fat cells, you'll have them for life. When you
lose weight, they shrink—at least temporarily. But then, thanks to a
fat-storing enzyme called lipoprotein lipase (LPL), they may stretch
out again, as if to say, "Look here, I'm empty. Come fill me up!"

Though fat cells can puff up slowly over the years, you often
gain new cells in "spurts." Two predictable spurts in childhood
occur shortly after birth and between nine and thirteen years of age.
Other spurts tend to occur during times of great change and stress
in our lives, such as when we leave home, during pregnancy, while
going through menopause, or after enduring a life-threatening
emotional trauma, such as being raped. Many women report gaining a bundle of weight after being promoted or while going to graduate school.

Your multiple kinds of fat cells differ by more than just color,
size, and location. They also have many different "receptors," like
little locked doors, that respond to specific hormones, which act
like little keys. Your fat cells constantly bathe in hormones like catecholamines and cortisol (your stress hormones) and estrogen, progesterone, and testosterone (the sex hormones). But each little door
on each fat cell responds to only one hormonal key, and different
kinds of fat have different doors. By locking and unlocking different
doors on different cells, your various hormones determine which
cells will get the fat, how fast you'll store fat, and how fast you'll
release it. These are one-way doors. Some doors let fat into the
cells. Other doors let it out. Your fat cells can even add or erase certain doors. So, over time, these billions of smart little cells can

remodel or redesign themselves, becoming more or less responsive to different hormones.

I always envisioned my fat cells as lazy, slothful blobs just lying around in my body, sort of like a billion look-alike couch potatoes flopped before the TV guzzling beer. That's 100 percent wrong. Fat cells not only look quite different, but they're quite busily active. In response to hormone keys, your fat cell doors are constantly opening and closing, revving up or lowering your rates of fat release and fat storage.

The Unhealthy Fat

We're frequently told we're facing a dangerous "obesity epidemic," as if fat cells were all alike and equally deadly. But in fact, of these many different kinds of fat cells, only *one type* has ever been strongly linked to hypertension, heart disease, stroke, diabetes, and some forms of cancers. Which kind? The deep, "visceral" white fat located inside your abdomen around vital organs like your heart and liver.

All other fat—the brown fat, the white fat in your breasts, derriere, calves and so forth—won't seriously harm your health, unless you get so fat it's hard on your joints or you have trouble walking. Some fat, like that in your bottom and thighs, may even *protect* your heart. We'll talk much more about this new understanding in a minute.

The first scientist to observe that people with fat above their waists frequently went on to develop diabetes, heart disease, gallstones, and gout, whereas people with fat below their waists had none of these health problems was the French physician Jean Vague. He called upper-body fat "android obesity" because it was more common in men and lower-body fat "gynoid obesity" because it was more common in women. But he recognized that some men carry their fat below their waists, whereas some women have the more "masculine" pattern. Today we simply call the android pattern "apple fat" and the gynoid pattern "pear fat."

Vague's work was seen as brilliant when it came out in the 1940s. But it wasn't discovered *how* brilliant until the late twentieth century when CT and MRI scans became widely available in hospitals. Suddenly, doctors began turning their machines on the human body and looking inside. That's when they discovered a special kind of upper-body fat: the "visceral" white fat hidden deep in your abdomen, the kind you can't see from the outside. A recent explosion of research has now confirmed this deep fat around your vital organs is the only type strongly linked to hypertension, heart disease, stroke, diabetes, and some forms of cancer. Daily Hassles Fat, Depression Fat, Lazy Thyroid Fat, Anger Fat, Binge-Eating Fat, PCOS, Post-Trauma Fat, Night-Eating Syndrome, some (but not all) Post-Pregnancy Fat, and Medication-Caused Fat are all kinds of apple fat. It's the kind of fat that needs to be lost.

In an extremely thorough review on body fat and disease, citing 462 studies, obesity expert Ahmed H. Kissebah and research scientist Glenn R. Krakower in the department of medicine, division of endocrinology, metabolism and clinical nutrition at Froedtert Memorial Lutheran Hospital in Milwaukee, Wisconsin, convincingly showed it's apple fat (not obesity per se) that's the risk factor for metabolic problems and a host of diseases. All other types of fat are now considered metabolically harmless.

I was stunned to find this fact is so well established, it's almost not even worth debating.

In the old ways of thinking, unhealthy fat was measured in *pounds*. In the new ways of thinking, unhealthy fat is measured in *patterns*.

What makes the fat stored in your visceral cells so unhealthy? It's the only type of fat involved in a "tangled web" of metabolic disturbances known as the "Deadly Quartet" (high blood pressure, high triglycerides, high blood sugar, and visceral fat). This life-threatening syndrome, which has also been called the Civilization Syndrome or simply the Metabolic Syndrome, usually starts silently, then slowly progresses. Once one or more elements of the Deadly Quartet appear, any number of killer diseases may eventually follow. Among them: heart disease, stroke, adult-onset diabetes, gallstones, and breast or endometrial cancer. Under this new definition, even skinny people can be metabolically "obese" in the sense they have too much fat in their visceral cells.

It's crucial to add we're speaking here about the metabolic health of *fat*, not the mechanical difficulties that might develop from too much *weight*. It's important to make that distinction. For example, too much weight below your waist can put extra pressure on your knees and aggravate arthritis, but it's not going to give you a heart attack.

Does excess apple fat *cause* the rest of the Deadly Quartet? Nobody's sure. Since visceral fat cells are the most metabolically active kind of fat, they may promote the other elements of the quartet by rapidly dumping high amounts of free fatty acids directly into the liver. This precious organ does many critical jobs, including metabolizing drugs and detoxifying the body. When overloaded with fat, the liver can't do its jobs as well.

Still, it may not be apple fat itself that causes heart disease, diabetes, stroke, and other diseases. It may be other, confounding factors in our lives, particularly stress and the ways we attempt to deal with it (by smoking or drinking too much alcohol, for example), that cause both deep abdominal fat *and* major illness.

How Stress Causes Apple Fat

Since the late 1980s, a large and rapidly growing body of medical literature has linked chronic stress and its consequences (anger, depression, binge-eating, etc.) to high levels of upper-body fat, the rest of the Deadly Quartet, and a host of deadly diseases. "We know that the stress hormone cortisol coupled with adrenaline can drive fat to the abdomen," Duke University professor of psychiatry Redford B. Williams told me. "Stress actually seems to cause our bodies to redistribute our fat, relocating it from other areas, such as the thighs, to the tummy."

Okay, I'll buy that. But why doesn't all stress generate deep apple fat? Why don't *all* people subjected to stress develop the characteristic spare tire around the middle? Answer: genes play a role. So do sex hormones. But another important answer was provided by Swedish endocrinologist Per Bjorntorp. He has demonstrated that it's not stress per se, but how we react to it, that gives us the kind of unhealthy fat that's been linked to all those diseases.

Convinced that fat patterns can be altered not just by individual stressors (such as a divorce, poverty, or loss of a job) but also by broader stresses (such as earthquakes, hurricanes, and wars) experienced by an entire generation, Bjorntorp contacted all the men and women who had been born in one town in Sweden during the first six months of either 1944 or 1952. From the approximately 80 percent who responded, he then selected 284 men and 260 women based on their fat patterns and gave them full metabolic workups. In overweight people with intense cortisol responses, he found full-blown signs of the Deadly Quartet, including high levels of apple fat. But most revealing of all, these people were so chronically stressed that some had completely given up. In the most severe cases, perhaps 5 to 10 percent of the population, Bjorntorp observed a kind of "burnout." They'd been stressed by unrelenting demands and pressures for so long, their bodies and minds had succumbed to a kind of hormonal exhaustion. With no hope, they had given up searching for solutions. They could no longer respond to stress with any effort at all. "This is similar," Bjorntorp notes, "to the condition described as post-traumatic stress syndrome, as seen, for example, in army war veterans."

A study at Yale University tends to confirm Bjorntorp's findings Women who had high cortisol secretions when under stress and displayed a "powerless" or "defeated" reaction had more deep apple fat. They also reported frequently feeling that problems in their lives were beyond their control. Women who stored their fat in their hips and thighs, in contrast, did not have this powerless reaction. Even when they felt stressed, they still had the confidence to keep trying.

So does this mean all skinny people are superconfident and that if you have unhealthy fat, you cope with stress poorly? No. As you'll recall from the last chapter, we're all confident or insecure in different situations. Overweight people as a group have no more emotional problems than thin people do. On the contrary, some extra fat (especially in your hips and thighs) may even temporarily help you cope better with life's struggles. Whereas heavy people often eat when they're stressed, thin people cope with their emotional problems in other, often more dangerous ways: by smoking too much, becoming anorexic, or even committing suicide. Women sexually abused as children who develop Post-Trauma Fat may also have fewer post-traumatic stress symptoms later than those who become overly skinny. So some ways to be fat that at first glance appear to be unhealthy may really be healthy.

Sorting Out the Headlines

This new understanding—that it's not how fat you are, but *the kind of fat cells you have* and, more specifically, *where you store your fat* that determines whether it will lead to a killer disease—helps resolve a heated controversy that's been raging among scientists for many years. Since you're bound to hear remnants of this controversy in the popular press, we need to talk about it so you'll be able to take charge of your weight with less stress.

You'll often hear that gaining just 10 pounds after age twenty will shorten your life—and that losing those pounds will make you more healthy. This widely promoted claim has never been proved. In fact, among leading scientists, there has long been a firestorm of debate over how unhealthy being overweight really is. Even today, some researchers keep insisting that being "overweight"—20 to 30 percent or more over what's "desirable," according to the latest weight chart—will damage your health and lead to all sorts of diseases. With a few exceptions, scientists in this fear-all-the-fat camp tend to be rat researchers or epidemiologists who study broad groups of people (not individual humans). This highly vocal minority of scientists has dominated the public messages about fat for many years, at least in North America. But, in fact, their popularized health message—lose weight or die—has never been proved. As a well-publicized editorial in a January 1998 issue of the prestigious *New England Journal of Medicine* put it:

> Given the enormous social pressure to lose weight one might suppose there is clear and overwhelming evidence of the risks of obesity and the benefits of weight loss. Unfortunately, the data linking overweight and death, as well as the data showing the beneficial effects of weight loss, are limited, fragmentary, and often ambiguous.

Whereas some studies suggest being overweight goes hand in hand with poor health, others find being slightly overweight will actually help you live longer.

As I was trying to absorb all this and wondering whether I should order out for pizza, I stumbled on what's now become my all-time favorite study. It has a long scientific title, but I just call it the Fat Thighs Study. It was inspired by some scientists in the

Netherlands who asked an interesting question: Could it be that fat stored in safe spots like the thighs was better than "harmless," that it was actually healthy, acting as a kind of "metabolic sink" to drain off the bad effects of too much visceral fat? In other words, when it comes to your health, does your good fat cancel out your bad fat? Intrigued, a Stanford University team decided to check it out. First, they recruited 263 "moderately overweight," sedentary men and women by newspaper announcements, radio, and word of mouth. Then they measured their recruits' waists and thighs. Then they did blood tests to check their "healthy" HDL and "lousy" LDL cholesterol levels.

The result? Women *with the fattest thighs* had the best cholesterol profiles and the lowest risks of heart disease. Whew! Could it really be true? Could thigh fat somehow protect a woman's heart? It sounded preposterous. The Stanford team decided to double-check, just to make sure they were measuring *fat* and not bone or muscle. Sure enough, a closer look revealed it was thigh *fat* that accompanied better cholesterol levels. Still another astonishing study of 43,595 women reported in the *American Journal of Public Health* found overweight women with the widest hips also had lower rates of diabetes!

"We cannot say lower body [or pear] fat is totally harmless, particularly not in the extremes," says prominent Swedish obesity researcher Per Bjorntorp. After all, he notes, too much weight even below the waist can lead to varicose veins and trouble walking. Still, he adds, *moderately* heavy hips and thighs should be seen mainly as a cosmetic issue, much like a long nose, wide feet, or big ears. Or maybe we should just see thigh fat as sexy, the way Rubens did. I began eyeing my fat thighs as adorable lifesavers. You know, if you look at them just right, saddlebags *are* kinda cute.

So here we have yet another major puzzle. You've been hearing for years that being overweight is unhealthy. Yet another whole body of underreported research we'll get to in Chapter 7 ("Do You Have Healthy Fat?") shows being overweight *isn't* unhealthy, and overweight women often live *longer.*

Why? It all seems so perplexing. Why would some studies show that being overweight is unhealthy, while others show that it's not? Think about it a minute, and you can probably guess the answer.

To date, only some studies, such as the Fat Thighs Study, have taken into account the new understanding that there are many different kinds of fat, and only one kind—the apple kind stored in your visceral cells—is unhealthy. "Obesity" and "overweight" are continually misdefined and mismeasured as *how many pounds people weigh* when the vast majority of the most current research shows the true medical danger lies in *where people carry their fat.* The researchers haven't exactly been mixing apples with oranges. But they have been mixing apples with pears.

Until very recently, the studies linking fat to heart disease and other illnesses were also done almost exclusively on white, middle-aged *men.* Since apple fat is much more common in men, their excess "weight" (which pound-for-pound includes more apple fat) is much harder on their hearts than it is on ours. Compared to the typical male who carries his fat in his belly, however, a subgroup of individual men with fat thighs and big butts may be on the road to a ripe, robust old age. It depends on how much of their fat is in those visceral cells and how much is in safer storage compartments. (Unfortunately, this isn't easy to eyeball.)

Studies of huge populations also seldom, if ever, control for many of the most common contributors to deep abdominal fat, including smoking, alcohol, daily hassles, trauma, anger, depression, lack of exercise, medications, PCOS, thyroid problems, and all the other unhealthy ways to be fat. Large population studies obscure so many individual differences, in fact, it's impossible to say what they mean. Was it really *fat* that was linked to disease—or some other confounding factor like stress, depression, an underactive thyroid gland, or antidepressants that the study design didn't even consider?

The only good way to measure visceral fat is by looking deep inside the abdomen with a CT or MRI scan. The size of people's waists is a fairly good measure for broad groups of people, but it's not much good for unique individuals like you and me. (That's why you can't simply measure your waist with a tape measure and determine for sure how much visceral fat you're toting around.) Once population researchers begin separating people with healthy fat from those with unhealthy fat—once they start controlling for the multiple ways to be fat and stop viewing all overweight people as exactly the same—many seemingly contradictory findings about fat and our health will no doubt be resolved. Once it's fully realized in all medical circles (not just in the most well-equipped obesity labs) that some fat patterns are healthy while others are unhealthy—and that scientists on *both* sides of the debate have been partly right— the angry shouting matches over the hazards of all fat will subside. When the fat warriors finally declare a truce and the diet wars end, the relatively recent notion that all excess weight should be declared a "disease" will be seen as a short-lived medical fad.

But this inevitable growth in understanding won't happen over-night. In the meantime, you'll probably continue to see headlines screaming that all fat is deadly. When you do, just relax and take all that high-sounding rhetoric with a grain of salt. (Better yet, with a soothing cup of green tea.) The public debates over the dangers of fat that keep surfacing in the press are far more important to medi-cal technologists arguing over their research techniques than they are to you as a unique individual. Superconfident winners have replaced the goal of being thin at all costs with the goal of good health, and the only kinds of fat cells that can damage your health are the visceral kind. Next question: How do they get there?

CHAPTER 6

How You Form Unhealthy Fat Patterns

Your health is bound to be affected if, day after day, you say the opposite of what you feel, if you grovel before what you dislike and rejoice at what brings you nothing but misfortune. Our nervous system isn't just a fiction. It's a part of our physical body, and our soul exists in space and is inside us, like the teeth in our mouth. It can't be forever violated with impunity.

—Boris Pasternak,
Doctor Zhivago

Since the only unhealthy body fat is the kind deep in your abdomen, how do you collect this type of fat? Suppose you've just eaten a Belgian chocolate. Why would your body stash any given molecule from that chocolate in one of your visceral cells as opposed to a cell in your thigh?

The answer: it all has to do with hormones. Hormones are the doormen that unlock your fat cell doors so the fat can go in. In women, unhealthy fat patterns are formed mostly by stress hormones and a special response to stress we touched on briefly in the last chapter and will explore more fully in a minute. But first we need to dispense with two red herrings: calories and carbohydrates. These two confidence busters, which *don't* determine your fat patterns, can slow your progress so much you'll give up in defeat. They've sidetracked many women for years.

Why Calories Aren't the Answer

We live in a complex, ever-changing world, filled with stress, down-sizing, threats of poverty, fear of violence, and lack of meaning in our lives. We have genetically diverse bodies continually surging with hormones. We're all growing older, getting married, having babies, changing jobs, getting divorced. And in the midst of this constant change, we're frequently given only one narrow, rigid option for slimming down: eat less, exercise more. Is this prescription the magic bullet for all women? Well, let me ask you this: Has it worked well for you? If it has, why aren't you thin?

In fact, when it comes to gaining or losing unhealthy fat, calorie counting is surprisingly useless. Calories are merely units that measure energy, much as seconds measure time. Calories can't choose your fat patterns or be stored in your fat cells any more than seconds can choose the time of day or be stored in your wristwatch.

Calories are a fairly good weight-gain predictor in rats. But human studies have continually shown that overweight women as a group *eat no more and sometimes eat even less than slim women do*. You may have suspected this all along, but I was stunned when I first began reading it. I spent many afternoons in a medical library, poring through study after study, my mind reeling at this realization. Still, it's absolutely true. In a now-classic study published in the *British Journal of Nutrition*, scientists took a bunch of women and paired them up, so each pair was matched for weight, age, height, and daily activity levels. All these women had long maintained their weights on the amounts of food they were eating. These amounts were then measured over the next several weeks. When the amounts of food were examined, one member of each matched pair was often eating *twice* as many calories as the other. The same findings were also true for matched pairs of men.

Scientists have done everything they can to catch fat people in the act of eating more than thin people do. They've had fat and thin people make out food diaries. They've gone into restaurants and watched what fat and thin people eat. They've gone into fat and thin people's houses and peered into their cupboards and refrigerators. And they simply cannot catch fat people eating more. In *Annals of Behavioral Medicine*, University of Minnesota researchers Meena Shah and Robert W. Jeffrey summed up the results of more than half a century of research: "Reviews of research on the relationship between energy intake and obesity published up to the mid-1970s have generally concluded that there is *no conclusive evidence to support the idea that the obese consume more calories than the lean.* The present paper updates these previous reviews by examining new studies on this topic published since 1974. Twenty studies on this topic were located. . . . *Overall they confirm earlier findings.*"

In a study reported in the *New England Journal of Medicine,* people who considered themselves "diet-resistant" strongly believed their obesity was due to factors other than overeating. "Insofar as there were several causes of their problems," the editors of this prestigious medical journal conclude, "they were probably right."

We're often told that if we consume 3,500 calories more than we burn, we'll gain a pound. True? No. Why not? Because we all have different metabolisms. In one particularly ingenious study, Claude Bouchard and a team at Laval University overfed twenty-four male twins exactly 1,000 calories a day for eighty-four days, for a total excess of 84,000 calories per man. If gaining one pound were "simply" a matter of overeating 3,500 calories—in other words, if one pound = 3,500 calories—then each of these men should have gained *exactly* twenty-four pounds (84,000 divided by 3,500). But they didn't. Since they were twenty-four unique individuals, they gained anywhere from 9½ to 29 pounds. Some men gained *three times* more than the others on exactly the same diet! Bouchard also reports that individuals vary dramatically in their responses to exercise. Some people (especially men) can exercise, eat whatever they please, and lose weight. Others are so exercise-resistant he calls them "nonresponders."

Dieting by cutting calories—the very strategy that we've been told will "cure" fat—can wreck your metabolism so much you'll gain weight. In one classic study, as overweight women began shedding pounds, their resting metabolic rates fell by a whopping 28 percent. By the end of the study, "successful" dieters were burning fewer calories a day than naturally thin women, even though the dieters still weighed 60 percent more! On the many diets I tried, I'd lose weight for a while, then "plateau." Why? Because after you've cut calories for a while, your body rebels. Being no dummy, it protests, "I don't want to starve to death." So it slows down your metabolism to make sure you stop losing weight. And you do.

C. Wayne Callaway observes that *undereating* can alter a woman's metabolic rate and water balance to the point where she is literally starving and gaining weight at the same time. He says, "I continually see women in my practice who have dieted so much they can gain weight on a thousand calories a day."

Your body has so many tricks to slow down your metabolism it's impossible to outsmart them all. Factors that can raise or lower your metabolism include getting up or sitting down, time of year, time of day, time of month in your menstrual cycle, pregnancy, stress, medications, when you eat, how much you eat, even how deeply you *breathe*. We're sometimes advised to measure our metabolism. On what day? At what hour? So many variables affect your metabolism at any given moment on any given day that trying to measure the number of calories you're burning is like trying to measure a six-year-old's height as she's bouncing up and down on a pogo stick.

About all we can say about calories is that if you eat a bunch of them (more than your *individual* body happens to burn but not necessarily more than your sister eats), you will gain some fat. But how much you'll gain is anybody's guess. And where you'll gain it is determined by your hormones, not by how much food you eat. Calories can't choose your fat patterns.

The old calories in, calories out, idea wasn't totally *wrong*. It was right as far as it went. It was just too narrow and mechanical to explain why people gain unhealthy fat. It didn't go far enough. That's why the new thinking about fat is so important and so desperately needed.

Limiting Carbs Isn't the Answer, Either

You'll often hear that carbohydrates are a dieter's worst nightmare and even that carbs "make you fat." Is that true? No. Of the three food elements—fat, carbohydrates, and protein—only one type can be stored in your fat cells. Want to take a wild shot at which type? You're right. Fat. Scientists once thought humans could convert carbohydrates into fat, the way rats can. But we can't. As you may recall, when I first started my "Flatten Your Tummy" story, Harvard's George Blackburn told me that even if I ate ten thousand carrots, I would never store those extra carrots as fat. He said: "Rats can turn carbohydrates into fat. But humans can't. It's physiologically impossible"—and he's right. A very, very tiny amount of energy in fat cells comes from glucose (which, in turn, comes from carbs). But it's such a minute amount it's not even worth talking about.

So if carbs can't be squirreled away in your fat cells when you eat too much pasta or bread, where do the extra carbs go? To your liver and muscles, where they're stored as glycogen, the body's "preferred food." If you have glycogen in your system, your body will burn that before it dips into your fat stores. This is why when you cut out the carbs, particularly starches and sugar, you start burning fat sooner and keep burning it until you eat more carbs. But a diet that's too low in carbs (especially the important ones like fruits and vegetables) can cause major health problems. Besides, carbs can't choose your fat patterns.

Sex Hormones and Genes Play a Role

Okay, so let's go for the gold. If neither calories nor carbs can choose your fat patterns, what does? Certainly sex hormones play a role. The female hormones estrogen and progesterone like to store fat in healthy places like your hips and thighs, because their keys fit those doors. These "feminine" cells are bigger than those in your abdomen, and they hold onto their fat harder. So there *is* such a thing as a female fat cell (sorta). But you don't want to "outsmart" it, because it's healthy. If you strain to shrink healthy cells, how smart is that?

The male sex hormone testosterone, in contrast, likes to store fat in the visceral danger zone. In one telling study done in the Netherlands, ten slender young transsexuals undergoing sex-change operations were given extra testosterone in their transition from women to men. They not only acquired lower voices and more body hair, they also developed more visceral fat. After three years on testosterone, they had paid a steep price to leave womanhood behind: their visceral fat stores had increased 47 percent. In an opposite effect, men were given estrogen drugs to treat prostate cancer. As a surprising side effect, the fat cells in their bottoms got fatter. After menopause, when women's estrogen levels drop, we also tend to store more fat in our visceral zone. Even if we don't gain weight, our hormones may *redistribute* our fat, storing more of it around our middles.

Genes also determine how much visceral fat your body will store. Identical twin brothers are six times more likely to have the same fat patterns than men who don't share the same genes. Race also matters. Black women store less fat in their visceral cells, on average, than white women do. In one U.S. study at the Beltsville Human Nutrition Center and National Institutes of Health, scientists compared levels of visceral fat in black women and white women. Both groups weighed the same, had the same waist and hip sizes, and even had the same overall percentages of body fat. But when scientists turned their CT scans on these women, black women had 23 percent less fat in their visceral danger zones. What's more, black women continued to have less visceral fat even after both groups of women lost an average of 38 pounds. This finding helps explain why extra weight has seldom been strongly linked to heart disease in black women and provides a compelling reason for health policymakers to avoid applying Caucasian norms to all races.

Fortunately, although genes play some role in our fat patterns, biology is not destiny. The genes that make you fat are merely *susceptibility* genes, a set of options. You still have to make certain choices before you'll become fat in this particularly unhealthy way.

The Real Villains: Your Stress Hormones

You may think stress only makes you overeat. But there's far more to it than that. Hidden from view in your bloodstream, the hormones from your two stress systems can give you more unhealthy fat—even if you don't consume any more calories.

Two stress systems? That's right. Most of us think we have only one stress system—the fight-or-flight system. But in fact we have two. The first system—the sympathetic nervous system—releases the catecholamines that dissolve fat. The second—the hypothalamic-pituitary-adrenal system—releases cortisol, which stores fat in your visceral cells. They're both coordinated by structures deep in your brain, and both involve hormones released by the same glands (the pituitary and the adrenals). For years, doctors thought they were the same system, but they're not. They're activated by two separate endocrine highways and two different mental attitudes. As you go through your hectic day, on a level *below your awareness*, you're constantly turning these two stress systems on and off. By *consciously* learning to control these systems by becoming superconfident, you can rev up fat release and limit fat storage.

Right now, if you have a lot of unhealthy fat, that's a strong sign you spend much of your day in the low-confidence or "unhealthy-fat-storage" mode. One secret to weight-control victory is learning how to spend a lot more of your time in the superconfidence, "fat-dissolving" mode. So let's examine these two stress systems more closely.

Your Fat-Dissolving System

Your first stress system, your sympathetic-adrenal-medulla system, is the one that breaks down fat. It starts in a part of your brain called the amygdala, which relays messages on to the hypothalamus, a tiny part of your brain about the size of a small prune. The center of both emotionality and appetite, the hypothalamus tells you when you're hungry or full, hot or cold, stressed or calm. It responds to the way you interpret a situation. If you're feeling happily challenged or tense but still trying (that is, you're confidently making an effort), the hypothalamus begins revving up your body to act. It does this by sending a message on to the pituitary gland, telling *it* what to do.

Dangling from the hypothalamus "on a stalk like a cherry," the pea-sized pituitary (the body's master gland) then sends a message on to your adrenal glands, which sit perched like twins, one on top of each kidney. The inner core of these glands, or the medulla, then releases chemicals called *catecholamines*: epinephrine (also called adrenaline), norepinephrine, and dopamine. Also known as "the fight-or-flight hormones," catecholamines prepare your body to act when it's under threat by revving up your blood pressure, heartbeat, and breathing. They're also the only hormones in the human body that strongly affect the dissolving of fat.

Catecholamines release fat from your cells by locking onto four little "doors" (or receptors) on the cell's surface. Three of these doors (the beta receptors) stimulate fat release, and one door (the alpha receptor) slows it down. So, paradoxically, these hormones can both speed up fat breakdown and slow it down. They're a double-edged sword.

Catecholamines work so well at dissolving fat, they were one hidden ingredient in the diet-drug combination fen-phen. Unfortunately, chronically elevated levels of these stress hormones can also lead to heart disease. (This may be why some women on fen-phen suffered heart-valve damage.)

Catecholamines release unhealthy apple fat a lot faster than they release pear fat. There are four times more catecholamine doors on your apple-fat cells than on your thighs. This is why it's easier to lose inches around your middle than around your hips.

When you're releasing lots of catecholamines under stress, you're rapidly releasing fat from cells all over your body, but apple fat is being broken down fastest. If all the fat in your bloodstream doesn't get used and burned up to "fight or flee," it goes back into your fat cells for another day. So which cells get the fat at this point? If you've been straining so hard your confidence is shot and cortisol has kicked in, the fat you didn't use will be restored around your middle, even if it originally came from your bottom. Over time, if you're constantly under stress, you can literally *redistribute* your fat from your pear to your apple cells.

Your Fat-Storage System

Once you're so stressed you just want to throw in the towel, your second stress system—the cortisol highway, scientifically known as the hypothalamic-pituitary-adrenal system—kicks in. Cortisol, the "no-confidence" hormone, opens the doors to store fat. People with a lot of cortisol may also have a lot of Anger or Depression Fat. Chronically flooded with the no-confidence hormone, they may feel, "Why try? Nothing I do matters anyway." Deep abdominal visceral cells (the kind you can't see) have four times more cortisol doors than the fat cells right under your skin (the kind you can pinch).

Why does cortisol prefer to store fat in your visceral danger zone? It may be the way we evolved in the wilderness to get away from danger. Deep abdominal fat, being closest to the liver, is the fat you can mobilize most quickly during an emergency. If you're often in a state of red alert, your body may keep lots of visceral fat in storage so you can draw on it to fight or flee whenever you need it. By being stressed out a lot, you're telling your body, "Keep me fat. I need lots of reserves here to cope with all this danger."

Cortisol works with other chemicals to store fat faster and make fat cells larger. It can even deliver a quadruple whammy by raising your testosterone levels. In men, high cortisol levels lower testosterone. But in women, high cortisol levels make testosterone climb.

Other factors that can raise your cortisol levels include:

- Cortisol-containing prescription drugs. Drop-for-drop, the corticosteroid drug prednisone, for example, is five times more potent than the body's own cortisol, and many women gain weight when they're on it.
- Cigarette smoking. Heavy smokers have more visceral fat. More than thirty minutes after smoking just one cigarette, a smoker's cortisol levels are still elevated. We tend to think smoking reduces stress and keeps women *thin*, because it can raise body's metabolism about 10 percent. Yet in one study of nearly two thousand smokers over age fifty, the leanest people were those who lit up the *fewest* cigarettes (ten or fewer a day). The more cigarettes people puffed, the fatter their abdomens became.
- Alcohol. Alcoholics have chronically elevated cortisol levels and also high amounts of visceral fat. In one Swedish study, alcoholic men carried 48 percent of their body fat in their visceral cells, compared to 38 percent for teetotalers.

When your cortisol highway is working normally, Sweden's Per Bjorntorp explains, you're in excellent health. When this same stress pathway becomes hypersensitive, it can lead to a cascade of metabolic disturbances that can throw many hormones out of balance and lead to disease. Post-Trauma Fat has been scientifically linked to cortisol-releasing stress. So have Anger Fat, Depression Fat, Daily-Hassles Fat, Binge-Eating Disorder, and Night-Eating Syndrome. Even Polycystic Ovary Fat, Lazy Thyroid Fat, and some cases of Medication-Caused Fat may be related to hypersensitive cortisol responses. Since overstressed humans frequently smoke, drink alcohol, take antidepressants or tranquilizers, and lead sedentary lives,

Bjorntorp originally gave the Deadly Quartet another name: he called it the Civilization Syndrome. In these days of high-school murders, misinformation overload, and road rage (an unrelenting "stress epidemic"), is it any wonder that we're also experiencing an obesity epidemic?

One day, as I was pondering all this, I thought, Wouldn't it be terrific if you could somehow tell your two independent stress systems apart, if you could know by how you *feel* whether you're releasing catecholamines and dissolving unhealthy fat or releasing cortisol and storing it? To my absolute amazement, as my search for answers progressed, I discovered you *can* know whether you're dissolving or storing fat, because scientists already *do* know how your two stress systems feel.

How Your Two Stress Systems Feel

The first scientist to document how your two stress systems feel when they're activated by your mind was the brilliant Swedish psychoendocrinologist Marianne Frankenhaeuser. In an influential paper published in 1983, she dubbed the catecholamines the *effort* hormones and cortisol the *distress* hormone. She then watched stressed-out people in action, focusing on two aspects of psychobiological arousal: *effort* and *distress*.

Effort without distress (catecholamines without cortisol, or fat breakdown without fat storage), she found, is "a joyous, happy state." In this superconfident state, you may still feel some tension, but your concentration is keen and your adrenaline's pumping. Your skills are roughly equal to the challenges you face, and your talents are neither underused nor overtaxed. Aware and alert, you're making a strong effort to master your problems, and you're operating at your peak. On a good day, you feel high, almost euphoric. Who needs to eat?

Effort with distress (fat breakdown *with* fat storage) is the emotional state most typical of our daily hassles. If you're working in a high-pressure or tediously dull job or trying to raise an unruly teenager, you'll probably feel effort with distress. You're straining hard but fear you'll never succeed. As the hormones from your two stress systems soar, you feel jittery, irritated, angry, and maybe a little depressed. Your confidence is low, but you're still pushing hard. This is when you're not only dissolving fat but also starting to store it in your danger zone. Time for a piece of pie or a sixth cigarette.

If you keep pushing on, driving yourself harder, you'll eventually reach a stage of *distress without effort* (cortisol without catecholamines). This state feels lousiest of all. It means, Frankenhaeuser observed, "giving up, feeling helpless." You feel bored, impatient, tired, and irritated. Your confidence is shot. So is your concentration. The battle's over. You're defeated. Time for a giant bowl of Ben & Jerry's Chunky Monkey, a whole box of Godiva chocolates, or a stiff gin and tonic. With your low-confidence hormone in full command, you have little power to resist. And what happens when you eat all that food? It goes right to your visceral cells.

The big factor that determines which stress state you'll feel, Frankenhaeuser found, is your sense of *control* over the situation. The low-confidence cortisol state erupts when you're upset but feel you have no control. Many situations in modern-day life—such as getting a root canal in the dentist's chair, witnessing a bloody car wreck, watching starving children on the nightly news, listening to a deafening jackhammer outside your office window, trying to reason with a teen who's on drugs, or being dressed down by your boss in a meeting—cause distress with no way to fight or flee. You just have to hang tough. These are all cortisol-producing (unhealthy fat-storage) situations.

Effort without distress, in contrast, emerges when you feel happily challenged, in control, and on top of the world. In this joyous, superconfident state, Frankenhaeuser observed, the cortisol system is "put to rest."

These findings combined with the new understandings coming out of endocrinology have profound implications. They mean your mind can both rev up fat dissolving (by activating your high-confidence *effort* hormones) and *at the same time* reduce distress fat storage (by turning off your low-confidence *distress* hormones).

What's so startling about this new understanding is the realization that your mind strongly controls where your fat will be stored. You can literally determine whether your fat will wind up in your unhealthy apple cells by the ways you think and respond to stress.

To a large extent, you can *choose* your own fat patterns! Of all the new insights springing from this new biopsychosocial understanding of fat, this is probably the most stunning.

Beliefs That Can Make You Fat or Thin

The strength of your belief in your ability to handle any given situation determines which of your stress systems will kick in. Typical fat-storing "cortisol comments" tend to sound like this: "They're asking too much of me," "This deadline is impossible," "I'll never make this work," "This whole project's a mess," "I was born fat; I'll die fat," "I have no options left," "Oh, hell, the day's shot. Let's go out and get drunk." In contrast, superconfident beliefs (the kind that put the cortisol system to rest) sound more like this: "This is tough, but I know I'll find a way somehow," "If I just keep at this, I'm sure things will work out," "No matter how hard things get, I can't give up hope," "Steady, diligent effort always wins in the end," "I always stay open to new ideas. That's how I find solutions other people miss."

Let's look now to see how *effort without distress, effort with distress,* and *distress without effort* play out in a real woman's life. Brenda manages an office-temp service in Boston. We've all had bad hair days. This is one of Brenda's typical "bad fat" days.

She usually gets up in the morning feeling confident or at least reasonably okay. Maybe she'll have a small breakfast, although she's never particularly hungry. Then she heads off for work, where the early-morning hours usually go well; she's accomplishing a lot and feeling challenged but also relaxed. *(Effort without distress.)*

Then as the day wears on, the pressure begins to mount. She begins pushing harder. As the stress builds, her anxiety soars. Emergencies seem to pour out of the woodwork. She begins getting agitated. By noon, she's usually so buried under with work she barely has time to grab a quick sandwich at her desk. What if she can't get all these orders filled? What if something goes wrong? As the threats mount, her stress hormones go on red alert. Her breathing gets shallow, her heart races, her blood pressure climbs. She keeps pressing on, driving herself harder. Her clients are making impossible demands, but she's determined to put out every fire. She's never been a shirker, and she's not about to start now. By 3 P.M., she feels like snapping angrily at every interruption. But she bites her tongue and keeps on plowing ahead. (*Effort with distress has been going on for some time.*) She's burning fat, but cortisol has also kicked in.

By the time Brenda leaves work and arrives home (late as usual), she's so blasted exhausted she just wants to flop in front of the TV. On the nightly news, a teenager has just shot up his high-school class with a semiautomatic, and a seven-year-old girl's raped and mutilated body has been found in the desert. She sighs. Reminding herself she has more paperwork to do, she flips off the tube. The nerve-frazzling angst of the day has burned itself out. Her confidence is shot. She feels tired, irritated, and drained. (*Distress without effort—unhealthy visceral-fat storage without fat breakdown—has now fully kicked in.*)

After being tough and in control all day, she feels like giving herself a break. She deserves it. Heading for the kitchen, she eats seventeen chocolate cookies (seventeen, count them!). Or half a pound of Brie. Or a quart of ice cream. (*At this point, with her body full of cortisol, much of the fat from her snack will be stored in her visceral cells.*) Afterward, she mercilessly berates herself: "I can't believe I ate all that. How can I be so stupid? I have absolutely no willpower. Why do I do these awful things to myself?" Feeling fat and totally out of control, she makes a few halfhearted stabs at that paperwork, then gives up and goes to bed in a funk. Tomorrow, she swears, will be different. Tomorrow, she'll stay in charge.

Unfortunately, Brenda has a full-blown case of Daily Hassles Fat, complicated with some Binge-Eating Fat, Depression Fat, and Anger Fat thrown in. Until she can boost her confidence enough to handle her stressful life better, that spare tire of hers will continue to grow.

Okay, we've seen now how unhealthy fat develops. But what about healthy fat, the kind *not* linked to distress? That's a good question. In fact, before you can decide whether you want to work hard to slim down, you need to decide whether your fat is healthy or not.

CHAPTER 7

Do You Have Healthy Fat?

There are two sides to every question.

—*Protagoras*

Several years ago, I met a woman named Cindy in the locker room at the gym where I used to swim. I never learned her last name. But, as you probably know, when women undress together, they chat a lot. The more clothes we shed, the more we shed our false selves. At such moments, it's easy to tell a relative stranger your most intimate secrets.

Cindy was in her mid-thirties with an infectious, spontaneous laugh and curly, sandy-blond hair. She had many secrets about a man she was dating and a job she was about to leave. But her biggest secret was this: she weighed 185 pounds.

How could *that* be a secret, you ask? It was a secret because she looked about 150, maybe even 140. She must have had a body like a rock. She could swim a mile probably twice as fast as I could. She was like a torpedo shooting down that lane. She told me she also walked miles and miles every week just because she loved walking so much.

Yet despite her high energy, Cindy was extremely ambivalent about her weight. On one level, she felt confidently vigorous, assuring me that all the women in her family were heavy, and her grandmother was still a paragon of health at age ninety-three. On another level, she felt fat and thought she needed to lose 20 pounds. She was half-convinced that if she were only thinner, her new boyfriend would marry her in a minute. Yet she was strong and independent enough to wonder whether a man with such superficial standards was really worth keeping.

If I knew then what I know now, I would have suggested that she keep the weight and dump the man. Cindy was certainly no sylph. *Vogue* won't be calling her anytime soon. But when she wasn't worrying about her size, she exuded a sense of calm, confident power. She was one of those strong women in our fear-all-fat culture that diet gurus never mention: women who are both heavy *and* healthy.

Could it be that your fat is healthy? It's an important question to ask. In one recent University of Massachusetts survey, 47 percent of white women and 25 percent of black women were trying to lose weight—primarily "for their health"—when they weren't even overweight. Since you can't see the fat in your visceral cells (it's too deep inside your abdomen to eyeball), how can you figure out how much you're toting around? Aside from getting an expensive CT or MRI scan, here are six steps that will help you determine whether your fat is healthy.

STEP 1: LOOK IN THE MIRROR

This is the least accurate method, but it can be a useful first step. A good, long look at yourself naked in a full-length mirror will tell you in an instant whether you're an apple (carrying a lot of fat around your middle, where it could be unhealthy) or a pear (carrying the bulk of your fat in your thighs and hips, where it's healthy). Look at yourself from the front, then from behind. Try to do this in a warm, accepting, self-loving way. If you're apple-shaped, your fat could *still* be healthy if you're carrying most of it in the cells right under your skin (the kind of fat you can pinch). So this isn't a definitive diagnosis. It's only a starter. Still, it's a clue. (If you can't bring yourself to do the mirror test without cringing, consider whether you have body-image problems you want to address before you try to lose weight.)

STEP 2: FIGURE YOUR WHR

A more accurate measure of deep visceral fat is your waist-to-hip ratio (or WHR). Simply dig out a tape measure. Then divide your waist measurement (at its narrowest) by the distance around your hips (at their widest). A woman with a 27-inch waist and 38½-inch hips has a WHR of 0.70. According to C. Wayne Callaway, who has been very influential in drawing up U.S. government guidelines, a

WHR over 0.80 (assuming you're a woman) indicates you may need to lose that paunch.

You may also be able to get a rough estimate of your visceral stores simply by measuring your waistline. "According to NIH recommendations, there's trouble brewing when your waist is 35 inches or more (40 inches or more in a man)," says National Institute on Aging clinical director Reubin Andres, M.D. In addition, he notes, the World Health Organization has delineated a sort of "gray zone" when you should be "maybe a little concerned." As a woman, you cross into this gray zone when your waist reaches 32 to 34 inches (in a man, it's when his belt size becomes 37 to 39 inches).

What about those weight charts we see all the time? Is the body mass index (BMI) a good measure of unhealthy fat? No. Weight charts by their very definition measure only *weight*, not *fat patterns*. So they're virtually useless for determining the amount of fat in your visceral cells. According to Claude Bouchard, executive director of the Pennington Biomedical Research Center at Louisiana State University, you can take two people of exactly the same height and weight. The first person's body might be only 15 percent fat. The second's body might be 41 percent fat. In other words, you could weigh more than the woman next door and still have less unhealthy fat than she does. Even a skinny woman, especially if she smokes, never exercises, and drinks lots of alcohol, may have more visceral fat than you do.

The WHR and waist measurements are better measures of unhealthy fat than weight charts because they at least take into account the existence of fat patterns. But, even so, WHR and waist size are just a beginning. You need to go further.

STEP 3: FACTOR IN YOUR AGE

Being fat and staying that way can be much harder on your heart if you're thirty than if you're eighty. Why? Because "young fat" is more metabolically active than "old fat," and it has more years to do hidden damage. As you get older, a little extra fat can also protect you if you ever get a serious disease like cancer. Conversely, if you're pencil-thin at eighty, a vicious flu epidemic could do you in.

Are there any fat eighty-year-olds? Sure. Look around. You'll see them everywhere. A researcher in Boston who studies centenarians is fond of saying, "There are no fat one-hundred-year-olds."

But that's simply not true. I once saw an exceedingly plump (even "obese") guy on TV who was 109 years old. He was laughing, chomping a hot dog, and having a ball at Disneyland.

The reason you see so few really fat old people is this: for the first two-thirds of our lives, we tend to gain weight fairly easily. But from age sixty-five or so on, we begin to *lose* weight (on average). After sixty-five, the normal and more deadly trend on the scales is downward. If you're approaching eighty and you're still fat and feel great, more power to you.

STEP 4: FIND OUT YOUR NUMBERS

If you think you may have too much visceral fat, go to your doctor and have a full metabolic workup. See if you have any signs of the Deadly Quartet. If you do, you may be on the road to a heart attack, a stroke, diabetes, or some forms of cancer—and being overweight only worsens your odds.

Have your doctor order three tests: a fasting glucose test, a triglyceride (or blood fat) test, and an HDL cholesterol test. These tests should all be taken in the morning before you've eaten. In fact, you should eat nothing after 8 P.M. the night before. Your "fasting" glucose level should be lower than 110, your triglycerides less than 150, and your HDL above 45 or 50 (higher is better).

After these tests are taken, a second glucose tolerance test should be done one to two hours after you drink 75 grams of glucose. The results of this test should be lower than 140. If all your numbers are fine, your blood pressure is below 140/90 *and* you're a pear, these are good signs your fat won't give you a heart attack. Still, there's one more factor to consider.

STEP 5: LOOK AT YOUR FAMILY TREE

Do you come from a family of "big women" who live long, healthy lives? Doctors once thought that hereditary diseases were limited to rare maladies like hemophilia or certain birth defects. But ongoing research indicates nearly all ailments—including heart disease, breast cancer, diabetes, and hypertension—have some genetic component. How much your risk increases when a close family member has an ailment varies with the disease. According to a University of Utah School of Medicine study, if you're under age fifty and two or more close relatives have had coronary heart disease, your risk is three to six times higher than normal. If they had the disease early in life (before age fifty-five), your chances jump to four to thirteen times the average. That's not to say if a disease runs in your family, you'll automatically get it. But having a family history of heart disease if you're also fat greatly increases your odds.

So take a detailed family history. Most important to record: the health histories of your first-degree relatives—parents, siblings, and children—who have 50 percent of their genes in common with yours. Second-degree relatives—grandparents, uncles, aunts, nieces, and nephews—share 25 percent of your genes. Once you've taken a detailed family history, share it with your doctor. That moderately high blood pressure may suddenly become greater cause for concern if your mother, aunt, and grandmother all had heart attacks in their fifties.

STEP 6: CONSIDER YOUR LIFESTYLE

If you passed all the above tests with flying colors, here's the final test: How healthy are your everyday habits? Do you eat nutritiously (plenty of fruits, vegetables, and whole grains) and exercise regularly? If you answered yes to both, and you're a nonsmoker, drink alcohol moderately (if at all), have one or two dear friends you love laughing with, and feel your life is full of meaning, why are you reading this book? Forget about dieting. Go out and party. You're living a wonderful life. Your extra weight is *not* going to damage your health, and it may even help you live longer.

Losing Weight for Appearance versus Health

About now some of you may be thinking, "I don't care if my fat *is* healthy. I still want to lose it—if not for my health, just for my looks. Look at Julia Roberts. I'd die to look like that." Can you lose healthy fat—if you want to—just to look more terrific in the world's eyes and make all your rivals green with envy?

Of course. It may not be *wise* to lose healthy fat, but it's certainly *possible*. No fat, healthy or otherwise, is mysteriously glued into your cells. You need only to flip on the nightly news to see thousands of starving people who've lost healthy fat. I know your goal isn't to look like a starving refugee (or at least I hope it isn't). I'm only saying this to make the point that healthy fat is just backup energy in storage. Nothing more.

Since this book is about your taking charge, only you can decide whether you want to lose healthy fat just for looks. Only you can make this decision. To help you do that, however, here are some pros and cons to ponder:

On the plus side, there are some advantages to losing healthy fat. Many people may ooh and aah over you, saying you look terrific. People in your office may regard you as a paragon of self-denial and self-discipline. You can stride along the beach in a bikini. You may even earn more money by being fashionably thin, especially if you're in a trendy glamour profession like acting, modeling, or TV journalism. It's lousy that women are still judged and even hired based on how we look rather than on how competent we are. Still, this is a reality in the world. Until we change the world, this reality will keep cropping up. So on the benefit side of losing healthy fat, you have fashionable beauty, status, and prestige—goals you may have pursued all your life.

On the other side of the equation, straining to lose healthy fat has only one major drawback: it could shorten your life. Or, then again, it may not. The truth is, nobody knows. Some experts believe the human body was designed for feast or famine, that losing and gaining weight throughout our life cycles is perfectly normal. Others worry that too much yo-yoing or dieting to become super-thin could do you great harm.

In the First National Health and Nutrition Examination Survey (NHANES), women with body mass indexes (BMIs) between 26 and 29 who *lost weight* were 360 percent more likely to die from a heart attack than those whose weight remained stable. It's a startling finding. In plain English, it means a five-foot-four woman in this "probably-should-not-lose-weight" range would weigh somewhere between 152 and 170 pounds.

In the Iowa Women's Health Study of 33,760 women, it wasn't overweight women but those who *varied in their weights* who were most apt to die early. Women least likely to die from heart disease were those who had small weight *gains.*

Mounting evidence suggests it's only the extremes on the weight scale—being *much* too fat or *much* too thin—that lead to health problems. In one influential review of thirteen studies done by Ancel Keys at the University of Minnesota, the lowest death rates also went hand in hand with modest weight gains over the course of one's life. Noting that being too thin is just as unhealthy as being too fat and that weight had absolutely no impact on the middle 80 percent of women, Keys concluded, "The idea has been greatly oversold that the risk of dying prematurely or of having a heart attack is directly related to the relative body weight."

So the bottom line is this: some strong and mounting evidence suggests losing healthy fat could, indeed, damage your health, especially if you start yo-yoing. Dieting unnecessarily may also set the stage for binge eating. That's why it's so important to think through your weight-loss decisions carefully before you decide what you want to do. Risky practices like fasting for twenty-four hours straight, vomiting after eating, and taking laxatives, diuretics, or diet pills to lose fat should be avoided in any case.

On the other hand, if you now know you have unhealthy fat, it's time to begin taking it off. Let's start the process.

CHAPTER 8

Choosing to Take Charge

Everything can be taken from a man but one thing: the last of the human freedoms—to choose one's attitude in any given set of circumstances, to choose one's own way.

—*Viktor E. Frankl,*
Man's Search for Meaning

In every potential weight-loss winner's life, there comes a day, an hour, maybe just a brief moment when she's offered a choice: Will she continue down the road others have laid out for her, following *their* rules, and meeting everyone else's needs before she takes care of her own? Or will she strike out on what poet Robert Frost so eloquently called "the road less traveled," the road that leads to the authentic life only she can define? Whether she decides to stay at her present weight because it suits her or to slim down because that suits her even more, a woman destined to become a winner always chooses the second road, the one that leads to her own truths.

Lying in bed alone on a bleak November morning with snow blowing outside her window, Jill had no idea the new direction she was about to choose would eventually change her life. She felt compelled only to make a decision: Was the chance of recovering her health so hopeless she should just take an overdose of tranquilizers and end it all? Or should she keep trying? Lying under her cornflower-blue comforter, depressed to the point of suicide, every inch of her body longed to give up. But a deeper, stronger part of her kept saying, "You deserve better than this and you have three kids to support. Believe in yourself enough to keep searching for answers."

Jill's health had begun deteriorating rapidly two years earlier when her marriage was on the skids. Shortly after she went off birth-control pills (she was too angry at her husband to have sex), her periods became wildly erratic. She also started putting on colossal amounts of weight, gaining over 70 pounds in less than a year. "I got acne, suffered mood swings, and grew facial hair. Just like that—very rapid-fire. I'll never forget how mortified I felt one evening when I walked into the living room and my husband and a friend of his ridiculed me because I'd forgotten to clip the hair on my upper lip. They pointed and laughed, 'Oh, look, you're growing a mustache!' That night, I cried myself to sleep." Shortly after that, she filed for divorce.

Over the next two years, Jill's health problems escalated. "When I told my doctor how scared I was, he replied, 'You're just under stress.' His attitude was basically, 'Don't worry your pretty little head about it.'" When friends and relatives were equally unsympathetic, she became deeply depressed. "That's when my family doctor put me on antidepressants. Amitriptyline was his favorite. I hated that one. It turned me into a zombie. It would have me sleeping as much as eighteen hours a day. Here I was, now a single mother struggling to support three children, and I was so lethargic I could no longer work." Once a size six, she now weighed 185 pounds, and her blood pressure was soaring.

Lying in bed on that bleak November day, tormented with thoughts of suicide, Jill decided she deserved better. She needed to stop blaming herself for all the torments other people inflicted on her and start putting herself first for a change. She dragged herself out of bed, got dressed, and went next door to ask a neighbor if she knew any good doctors. Three days later, in her new gynecologist's office, Jill at last learned the real cause of her health problems, including her skyrocketing weight: she had Polycystic Ovary Syndrome, or PCOS, described by her doctor as "a genetic hormonal disorder, often triggered by stress."

Just knowing at last what was wrong gave Jill a great surge of confidence. The minute she got home, she made a beeline for the Internet to learn everything she could about PCOS. Over the next several months, with the help of an endocrinologist and medication, she got her hormones back in balance. Her acne and facial hair went away. She also started dieting and exercising again and lost weight.

Today, Jill is back to a size six, has a new public-relations job, and is dating a man who respects her. When people remark, "You look sensational!" and ask how she did it, she rattles off her regular spiel about PCOS, also describing what she eats and how much she exercises. But on a deeper level, she knows the real truth is much harder to put into words. What led to her strikingly obvious outer transformation took place invisibly in her mind on that bleak November morning, when she heard her true voice speak clearly for the first time and vowed to trust and follow her inner authority. It was during that split second when she realized she had always been stronger than she'd imagined, and she was worth the extra effort it would take to make her life work, that she took the first step toward redeeming her health. The unhealthy fat she lost was just a side effect of taking charge and learning what was really wrong with her.

When we see someone as healthy and happy as Jill, we might well ask, "Well, why can't I take charge like that?" When we have a choice in our lives between taking personal control versus relinquishing control and depending on others, why would any self-respecting grown woman choose the dependency route?

Overweight women often find it hard to take charge because confidence-sapping cultural messages continually brand them as "inferior" and unable to handle their problems. ("After all, if you're so competent," the unspoken message goes, "why are you fat?") "When people are cast in subordinate roles or are assigned inferior labels," Stanford's Bandura notes, "they perform at levels below their abilities." A kind of pseudo-incompetence sets in. If you're fat and have subconsciously bought into the societal message that you're "unattractive" and, what's worse, it's your fault, you may be unable to stick with the simplest eating and exercise plan. Just seeing an overweight woman walking down the street may make you doubt your own ability to slim down.

Still, if you've been unable to slim down, doesn't that mean you *are* incompetent in some ways? No. If you have healthy fat, your inability to lose it may be your body's way of protecting your health. Conversely, if you have unhealthy fat, there are two possible reasons why you've never taken it off: either you've never been told why you're fat, so you've lacked enough reliable information to get thin (a problem I'm hoping this book will help correct); or you have other priorities you subconsciously find more important.

Debbie is struggling with the second reason. On a conscious level, she's euphoric about having shed 46 pounds. But on a deeper level, being thin terrifies her. Why? Three years ago while crossing a parking lot after work, she was grabbed by three men, forced into the back of a van, and gang-raped. During the next year, she rapidly gained 53 pounds. Now, whenever she approaches the weight at which she was raped, she panics and quickly regains all the pounds she just lost.

Such past trauma is only one of many factors that can secretly sabotage your best efforts. Before you can take charge for life, you need to understand why you gained those pounds in the first place. Not *how*, but *why*.

By answering these three crucial questions, you can begin sorting that out.

1. WHAT DOES YOUR FAT MEAN?

Weight struggles may merely mean you're getting older or taking a fat-promoting medication. But as another possibility, fat may be helping you deal with distress.

On an unspoken level, you may have achieved a certain balance between the extra pounds you're carrying around and the overwhelming demands you're expected to meet. Many unpleasant situations in life seem almost impossible to control. At work, you may be handed catch 22–style problems to solve. You may be required to attend nerve-wracking business meetings, give impromptu speeches you're not ready to make, and go to business-related parties you find tediously dull. If you feel trapped at home, on the other hand, you may be so bored and unchallenged you just pig out all day. Overloaded by endless, routine chores, you may have barely enough energy left to wash your hair, let alone work out at a gym. With too little control over the rest of your life, it's easy to feel too little control over your weight. At the end of a harrowing day, it's hard to make smart decisions about your health when no one all day has asked what you thought or cared how you really felt.

Growth is hard. Going on single-magic-bullet diets and letting someone else tell us what to do may never make us thin, but it does keep us from having to make our own choices. As we look inside ourselves for the real reasons we've gained fat, we may find a deeper dissatisfaction with love, work, and our families than we ever expected, an anxiety that bathes every cell of our bodies. A haunting ambivalence about the choices we've made may surface: Why didn't I go to college when I had the chance? Should I have had children sooner—or not had them at all? Why have I stayed so long in this safe job when it's not what I want to do? Why did I marry this man? We may fear that we're "losing our edge" or that we have failed those we love most. Spiritual confusion may also erupt: What's the meaning of my life? Am I wasting my best talents? Was I put on this earth for a destiny I haven't begun to fulfill? When such questions arise, we can quickly push them out of awareness. We can think, instead, about food, our bulging tummies, or our fat thighs. But confusing questions that we fail to resolve earlier in our lives will keep surfacing again until we get them right. Avoiding the challenge now only means we'll have to face the same questions again later and accomplish less in the meantime. Denial of the search coupled with a whole bag of chips can relieve tensions temporarily. But they keep returning until that day when we dare to define our real values and find our most authentic selves.

Excess weight may offer many unexamined personal payoffs. What additional problems would you have to face if you were thinner? And here's a mind-twister: Since overweight women often cope better in emergencies than thin women do, how does your extra weight keep you sane or safe?

Gillian gained 35 pounds about three years ago at age fifty-four, when she was promoted to be a field investigator in child protective services in Atlanta. When she goes into a reportedly abusive home and often has to confront an angry parent twice her size, she has to make an instant decision: Is it safe to leave this child in this house at this time? If she's wrong in one way—if she takes the child away from a good-enough home—she has destroyed a family and traumatized a child. If she's wrong in the opposite direction—if she fails to observe clear danger signs and leaves the child in peril—the next phone call she gets may be one telling her the child has been murdered. Gillian doesn't drink alcohol, smoke, or take drugs. She doesn't drive cars too fast or sleep with dozens of men. At the end of a long, hard day, she just goes home and eats.

Are her cortisol levels frequently off the charts? Probably, considering all the horrors she sees. Has she ever thought about giving up her difficult job? "Absolutely not," she says, adamantly shaking her head. "These kids need me." Those 35 pounds she's gained over the past three years are the price she pays to care and keep caring. If we ever begin valuing women more for what they contribute to our society than for how they look, skinny actresses frolicking on movie screens will no longer be considered more "desirable" than impassioned caretakers like Gillian. Despite what the insurance charts say, Gillian may not really be "over" her ideal weight. On the contrary, she may have achieved her happy weight; she may be at exactly the right weight for her job (although by learning to handle her stress in less fattening ways, she can still slim down if she wants to).

We've already seen that not all overweight women overeat. But many of us do, especially when we're depressed, angry, or otherwise stressed. Here are just some of the more subtle unseen rewards winners report having to acknowledge before they could lose fat for life. See if any of them strikes a chord with you.

If I eat whatever I want, I may not permanently lose unhealthy fat, but:

- I can enjoy feeling out of control and breaking the rules without really rocking the boat.
- I can feel spontaneous and have fun for fun's sake without asking myself what I'd really love to do with my life.
- I can plead that I'm "too tired" to do tedious chores (or have sex) and then go to bed early.
- I can let my own feelings tell me what to do for a change instead of taking care of everyone else's feelings.
- I can blame my weight for the fact I feel my life is falling apart.
- I can be a martyr and show the world how much I can suffer with my head held high.
- I can be "difficult" and defiant and still not be branded angry or selfish.
- I can upset my fat-phobic mother and still pretend I'm being a "good girl."
- I can throw my weight around.
- I can feel comfortable walking through my dangerous neighborhood.
- I can stay faithful to my angry/boring/insensitive husband; if I ever lost weight, I'd probably have an affair.

Keeping unhealthy fat and avoiding change offers some benefits. Before some women are able to slim down for life, they need to face their ambivalence. Vincent J. Felliti, who heads a large weight program at a Kaiser Permanente group in San Diego, notes: "All the time in our program, we see people who on the one hand very much want to lose weight and on the other hand feel terrified—consciously or unconsciously—of the social and emotional consequences they'll have to face with any major weight change. What we've come to realize is that obesity very often is not the problem it's defined to be. Obesity is oftentimes somebody's *solution*."

Until you find different solutions, your fat may be hard to lose.

2. HOW OLD WERE YOU WHEN YOU STARTED PUTTING ON WEIGHT?

The question is not "When did you gain all the weight you have now?" but "When did the weight gain *begin*?" Was it after your parents got divorced, your mother died, or your car was rear-ended on the freeway? If you started gaining weight shortly after you started taking a medication, why did you need the medication? If it was an antidepressant, why were you depressed? The goal is to brainstorm until an answer makes sense. Why do you think you started gaining weight when you did and not two years earlier, or five years later? What was going on in your life? Did you just leave college and find it so hard to get a decent job you had to live in an unsafe neighborhood filled with muggers? Was your marriage on the rocks? Were you sexually harassed at work when you were just trying to do a good job? Did you have a crisis pregnancy? Did you suddenly begin working the night shift? (Some women say, "I was born fat." But that's not really true. No one is born fat. Newborns are never 30 or 40 pounds.)

Many women gain weight after a first, second, or third child when they begin working triple time to be loving mothers while also keeping house, trying to stay what society calls sexy, and paying their share of the mortgage. When women begin working what Arlie Hochschild called "the second shift," straining to juggle kids, career, and a husband, they often feel overwhelmed—and gain weight as a result of their daily hassles.

When Fat Signals Danger . . .

For some women, too much visceral fat (the submissive response) is a clear-cut physical sign of an underlying physical threat. Fat becomes a layer of self-protection, the only way the mind/body/spirit knows how to respond to a potentially life-threatening or emotionally painful situation.

If you're an overweight battered woman and need a safe place to hide (but have no one you trust), call a local crisis hot line in your area, or the National Domestic Violence Hotline at 1-800-799-SAFE for counseling or a referral to a safe house near you. If this number has changed for any reason, dial 1-800-555-1212 to see if you can get the new number. Until you can escape your abusive environment, unhealthy fat is the least of your problems and may even be your solution.

3. How's Your Support System?

Not long ago, a family doctor told me a story that brought home to me why some women want to stay fat. He described one of his diabetic patients, a 260-pound woman with high blood pressure and exorbitant cholesterol readings. Every time she came in, he nagged her to reduce. Finally, one day she told him the truth: "If I lose weight, I won't be as large, and my husband will start beating me up again. I'm terrified because he has a gun, and he's threatened to kill our two kids if I ever leave." Her doctor stopped pressuring her to go on a diet.

Plainly, achieving one's healthy weight requires having a healthy support system. It's hard to slim down if people keep sending you the message "We want you to stay fat. We're more comfortable with you this way." Richard Stuart, once a psychological director with Weight Watchers, tape-recorded dinnertime conversations between husbands and their overweight wives. The men mentioned food seven times more frequently than their wives did, offered the women food four times more often, and criticized their wives' eating behavior twelve times more than they praised it.

Wrestling with such secret sabotage, you may be fighting far more than your fat cells.

Victoria, married to a U.S. Navy ensign stationed in Norfolk, Virginia, was delighted to have lost 56 pounds. Shortly after she slimmed down, however, her husband began picking fights over everything from how she dressed to where she shopped for groceries. Victoria says, "After we fought nonstop for months, I realized he was far more comfortable leaving a fat wife on shore when he went out on tour than he was leaving a thin wife behind." She kept her figure, and her jealous husband adjusted.

In another survey by Stuart, virtually all the husbands of overweight women claimed they wanted their wives to slim down. Yet on another level, 38 percent said they feared a divorce if she did, 30 percent worried she'd have an affair, and 49 percent fretted they'd lose their "bargaining power" during an argument. (An example of such power: when she complains about his overspending, he can complain she's too fat.)

Having a genuinely loving support system, in contrast, will help you build the superconfidence you need to lose weight. How? For one thing, being supported in your efforts makes it easier to exert effort without distress. So in a very real way, the psychology of being loved affects the biology of your fat cells. For another thing, genuinely loving friends and family can give you happy boosts just when you need them most. Rather than "surprising" you with a gallon of your favorite ice cream, they'll bring home daisies or a book of poetry to show you their love, because they know you're struggling with your weight, and it's not easy.

Unfortunately, it's hard to break abusive family patterns. Ironically, the more abusive a family system is, the harder it can be to leave. Marge is five-foot-seven and weighs 245 pounds. At age thirty-six, she's also still living at home with her two children, her depressed mother, and her angry, alcoholic father, who on occasion still threatens to beat her. Before she can even think about losing weight, she needs to carve out more independence by moving out and creating a real home for herself and her children. She needs a "safe harbor" where she can become who she was meant to be and regain her health.

Some women berate themselves mercilessly if they can't seem to muster the alleged "willpower" to slim down. But, the truth is, it's okay not to be ready. Taking some time first to gain clarity about your life is also a powerful choice.

Winners were once "full of cortisol," if you will. They were constantly full of low-confidence, visceral-fat-storing thoughts and feelings like "They're asking too much of me," "I'm all washed up," "I was born fat, I'll die fat," "I can't change, I'm trapped," and "I have no options left." With steady, diligent work, they've abandoned such self-defeating attitudes and have acquired superconfident thoughts and feelings like these: "This is tough, but I know I'll find a way somehow," "No matter how bad things look, I can't give up hope," and "I always stay open to new ideas. That's how I find solutions others miss."

The process toward becoming a winner is not smooth and continuous. True change does not progress, as we're often taught to believe, in an unbroken, step-by-step, linear way. Rather a winner's understanding of herself and her health builds up until it reaches a critical threshold, suddenly triggering a change. Many winners talk about a "click" in their minds—a sort of quantum leap in awareness—that occurred right before they took charge, when they switched from an almost blind faith in obsolete one-size-fits-all answers and became very curious about their own individual ways to be fat. From that moment on, a winner discards all the old, unworkable prescriptions and begins seeking new, more effective solutions.

Psychologists Susan C. Olson and Robert H. Colvin, who studied weight-loss winners at the University of Arizona, have dubbed this shift from depending on others to taking individual responsibility the "Little Red Hen" transition, "a time of awareness, rethinking, making hard decisions." Following the example of the spunky Little Red Hen, the woman finally tires of waiting for others to solve all her problems. She impatiently snaps, "Then I'll do it myself." And she does.

Observe Your Thoughts

Winners often report setting aside at least a few minutes each day to breathe deeply and sit in silent solitude. (Now that you know how reacting to stress makes you fat, you can see why this works so well and could help make you thin.) During their quiet times, winners often report using a technique that sounds similar to a Tibetan Buddhist practice called "mindful meditation." There's a reason this technique works so well that it's now used in some medical clinics: mindfulness and other relaxation techniques alter *that same part of the brain where the cortisol highway begins* (the hypothalamus). So by relaxing deeply, you're literally boosting your super-confidence hormones. Mindfulness can be summed up in four words: being in the moment. Eventually, with practice, anybody can master this skill; it can help you cut down hair-trigger stress reactions throughout the day.

Many excellent books on mindfulness have been written, from Jon Kabat-Zinn's *Full Catastrophe Living* to Thich Nhat Hanh's *Mindful Living.* So there's no need to go over all the techniques here. But to get just a taste of mindful meditation right now, simply lie quietly alone in a room with the lights dim and the door closed. You might want to put some soft music on the stereo or light a scented candle. If you can't seem to relax lying down (for some women who've been sexually abused, lying down brings up painful memories), that's fine. There's no right or wrong way to do this. Just sit in a comfortable chair and place your feet flat on the floor, or relax in any other way that feels best to you. As you meditate, here are four skills you'll want to master:

TOTALLY RELAX YOUR BODY

Darby, a cardiovascular technician who has been meditating for many years, told me she starts with what Kabat-Zinn calls a "whole body scan."

> I lie on the bed and relax as much as I can, taking a number of deep breaths. I start at my toes and concentrate on making them as relaxed as I possibly can. Then I move up to my feet, my ankles, my calves, my knees, and so forth until I've reached my head. I always pay special attention to my abdominal area, around my stomach, because that's where I carry a lot of my stress. I might work to relax that area of my body for as long as five or ten minutes. I also spend extra time on my shoulders and the back of my neck. I focus on making each part of my body feel very heavy, as if every bit of effort were drained from me and I'm totally limp. [Other winners report using the same technique but relaxing by making themselves feel "light as

a feather," or, as one put it, "like I'm floating on a pink cloud."]
When I finally reach the top of my body, I envision the last bit of
tension flowing out through a hole in the top of my head, sort of like
a volcano or a whale blowing its spout. [She laughs.] *Now*, I'm ready
to fix dinner! But you know what? I no longer want half a pizza. I'll
often decide to have something light like a shrimp salad, instead.

LET YOUR WORRIES GO

A second step in becoming "mindful" involves watching your
thoughts. Randi, a winner who lost 29 pounds, explains, "As I relax,
I don't try to change my thoughts. No thought is good or bad. I just
notice which ones come up. I examine them, almost from a distance, turning them around in my mind. Then I slowly, gently let
them go into the air. I picture my worries drifting away."

Another winner says, "In the silence, I see my worries dissolve;
they start as a heavy black cloud and drift away like a wisp of gray
smoke." Still a third winner says, "When I first start meditating, my
mind is like a messy room, all cluttered. So I just picture taking my
worries and stacking them one by one neatly in a pile. I like to think
of myself as doing a little mental housecleaning."

At times, certain critical voices may keep yammering at you.
They may even tell you that you "can't" meditate, you're doing it
"wrong," or that you're being "lazy" to just sit there "doing nothing" when you should be working. Those are the critical voices of
others, not the thoughts of your deepest self. Notice these critical
voices as if you were an observer on a far distant hill: don't take
them in. Just let them float through your mind, then let them go.
Over time, mindfulness becomes more than a way to relax. It
becomes a way of life. One day when the kids are crying, the dog's
barking, and the doorbell's ringing—or when you're in the middle
of a tense business meeting that's making everyone else's blood
boil—you'll find yourself stepping back deliberately from the fra-
cas, pondering the situation, dropping peacefully into a mindful
state, and thinking to yourself, "Wow! I can handle anything."

PICTURE YOUR PROBLEM

As they work to take charge of their weight, winners often observe
their thoughts about food and even "picture" their eating problems.

"Through silence, I learned a lot about my bingeing," says Nora, a visual artist who's now a happy 117 pounds. How? "Basically, I just called up my binge-eating problem and talked to it." How? She laughs. "Well, first of all, I should preface this by saying I'm quite imaginative. I have very vivid fantasies. Some people might think this sounds silly. But for me, it was fun and quite simple. First, I started daydreaming and asked myself, 'If my eating problem were an animal, what would it look like?' To my astonishment, a spider appeared in my imagination; it looked rather like a big, brown, hairy tarantula. A spider! Not quite an animal, but close. I was really shocked! So in my daydream, I asked this spider, 'What are you doing here?' And the creature replied, 'I feel really mean inside because you'll never let me be free.' That puzzled me awhile. But once I thought about it, I realized I often do feel 'really mean inside' when I binge. The spider was telling me I wanted to stop feeling bad and be free." After this insight, Nora began noticing more closely when she felt calmly loving inside and when she felt mean. Over time, she came to realize her "meanness inside" erupted mostly when she was pushing herself too hard, especially when she was on deadline. That's when she ate. The hassle-fat-reducing answer: she began giving herself more time to complete projects and a day off now and then. As she developed more patience, her food cravings lessened.

Sabrina, another winner, visualized her fat cells and asked why they always tormented her so. In her imagination, the "cells" replied, "We're not tormenting you. We're just a bunch of giggling little girls down here, having good fun." The deeper understanding she took from this message was that if she wanted to lose her unhealthy fat, she needed to give herself more fun that didn't involve food. Since she'd broken up with a longtime lover, she'd been terribly lonely and bored. She resumed watercolor painting (a talent she'd let slide), began flower gardening, took up playing the piano, and made friends with two fun-loving women at work who also wanted to "giggle." At last report, she'd lost 83 pounds.

ASK WHY YOU NEED STRESS

If you're a high-voltage Type A, you may find it very difficult to unwind enough to meditate. Lying quietly alone may only make you *more* tense. If you have this problem yet still feel constantly has-sled, you need to ask yourself why. Many women have difficulty giving up stress because on some level, it makes us feel more important. People are counting on us. We're in demand. We're needed. We can't let "them" down. Somewhere along the way, we have been sold a bill of goods: stressed people are Very Important People. We take a certain obstinate pride in being overextended.

In fact, there is a deeper self who truly *is* a very important person, not just to "them" (whoever those demanding others might be), but possibly to all of creation. This deeper self, always inside you, quietly watching the hullabaloo, doesn't emerge under pressure or deadlines. She unfolds and blossoms most when she's loved, cherished, and gently nudged to grow strong. The Watcher. You've felt her. She was there when you were born, when you were three, when you were twelve. She is there still. In the silence of your being, at the core, in the center, she is there, quietly watching, patiently waiting. The Watcher knows who you were meant to be. She carries with her a blueprint for your true self, for your healing. She will speak when she's ready. But you must be ready to listen. Now try again. Keep searching . . .

PART THREE

Be a Weight-Loss Winner

CHAPTER 9

Losing Daily Hassles Fat

The world can be divided into two types of people: The ones who stop eating under stress—and the ones who don't.

—Joel Yager, M.D., former director,
UCLA Eating Disorders Program

Leah, thirty-eight, is good at her job. As a customer-service rep for a large Boston department store, she always hangs tough while handling the avalanche of complaining customers who arrive at her counter. Still, after following the rules and smiling at angry people all day, she feels so frazzled by 6 P.M. that she could use a stiff drink.

Fortunately for her waistline, there's no time for that. She immediately heads for home, where her workday continues as she fixes dinner with one child crying, the phone ringing, and another child whining about doing his homework. After dinner, her husband, Bill, does the dishes so she can dash to the mini-mart to buy cereal for breakfast. Back home, she folds a load of laundry that's been in the dryer three days. By 9 P.M., when the kids have finally been bathed, read a fairy tale, and tucked into bed, she's exhausted and ravenously hungry. She deserves a break. She heads for the kitchen. Maybe she'll have just half a brownie. Or why not the whole thing? Ah, it tastes so good. It's comforting to do what *she* wants for a change. Her stress levels drop. Before she knows it, she's eaten every brownie on the plate. How many were there—three, four? Staring at the few remaining crumbs on the empty plate, she feels guilty but at the same time a little defiant and free. Hey, it's okay. Get back in control. Don't give yourself such a hard time.

You're strong. What's done is done. No need to whine. She washes the plate, then goes into the den and settles down on the sofa beside Bill, who's watching the news on TV.

Not surprisingly, Leah (who's five-foot-three) yo-yos between 140 and 160 pounds and dreams of being 120. So what makes her fat? At first glance, you might say, "Those brownies." But with a deeper, broader understanding, you can see it was really all those daily hassles that eventually did her in. Tomorrow morning she'll step on the scale as usual, sigh, and tell herself, "Damn! I'd be so much less stressed if I could just lose some weight." But her extra pounds are the *result* of her stress, not the cause.

Unfortunately, nobody leads a hassle-free life. For most of us, too much to do, impossible deadlines, lost car keys, maxed-out credit cards, pushy people, threats of layoffs, and traffic jams are just part of the usual routine. Because such irritations are ubiquitous, you may dismiss them as trivial. Yet hundreds and thousands of such minor irritants over months and years can give you Daily Hassles Fat. Elevated cortisol levels, which can lead to too much unhealthy visceral fat, have been found among supermarket cashiers with neck and shoulder pains; college students during midterms and final exams; women going through menopause; overwhelmed women trying to juggle careers, marriage, and children; women with premenstrual syndrome; women who've just lost their jobs; and those who only *fear* losing their jobs. Even watching the nightly news or a violent film can trigger high cortisol levels.

The more hassles you face, a University of California at Berkeley study found, the more you're also likely to develop ills like back and chest pains, headaches, stomach cramps, or high blood pressure. So here's how to develop the superconfidence to get those hassles under control. (These skills work well for all kinds of stress-related fat. So you may want to mark this chapter with a Post-it.)

Is This Your Problem?

1. Do you often feel distressed just while going about your daily routine?

2. Do you push hard all day, then almost fall into a stupor from exhaustion at night?

3. Do you frequently suffer from physical signs of stress, such as headaches, neck and shoulder pains, an upset stomach, insomnia—or a lot of visceral fat?

4. Do you tend to worry about "little things" that don't seem to bother other people?

5. Do you find yourself getting angry or depressed much more often than you'd like?

6. Do you drink alcohol, smoke, or numb out in front of the TV to escape from your problems?

7. Do you often feel your life is hopeless, you're out of options, and nothing will ever work out?

If you answered yes to most of these questions—especially if these problems erupt frequently—you're probably struggling with Daily Hassles Fat. If you answered yes to questions 5 and 6, and if you're *chronically* angry or depressed, you may have a full-blown case of Civilization Syndrome and also need to read the chapters on losing Depression Fat, Anger Fat, and possibly Post-Trauma Fat.

1. Notice Your Trouble Zones

Fortunately, when hassles strike, you're not helpless. You can reduce Daily Hassles Fat by choosing how confidently you'll respond. When anxiety, anger, or depression mount, slow down and observe what's happening. What time of day is it? What or who are you thinking about? What got you stirred up? If you were watching TV, what were you watching? How are you feeling right now? Resentful, envious, worried, humiliated? What comfort foods are you craving? Many winners keep detailed journals to record their most common Daily Hassles Fat promoters and how they develop.

Even if you don't eat the minute daily hassles erupt, be wary of times later in the day when you're tired and your defenses go down. To gain clarity about how being chewed out by your boss at noon can make you pig out at 9 P.M., take this quiz, adapted from a scientifically validated scale designed by Matthew M. Clark at Brown University. Dig out a pencil or pen and star those times when you're least confident about your ability to stay in charge:

When you're anxious (or nervous)
When you're depressed (or tired)
When you're angry or irritable
When you've experienced a failure
On weekends
When you have many different kinds of food around
When you're at a party
When you're around your favorite foods
When you have to tell others "no thanks"
When you feel it's impolite or rude to refuse a second helping
When others are pressuring you to eat
When you think others will be offended or upset if you don't eat
When you feel physically run-down
When you have a headache
When you have other aches or pains
When you feel physically uncomfortable
When you're watching TV
When you're reading
Just before going to bed
When you're happy

Now look over the situations you've just starred. These are your trouble zones, the no-confidence situations in which you need to brainstorm for confidence-boosting solutions. Jot down any other trouble zones you can think of (perhaps when you come home from a party at which you had a miserable time).

2. CULTIVATE NEW SKILLS

From the list above, choose just one trouble zone you'd like to work on. Have you ever been able to control your eating in this situation? If so, how? What skills did you use? What worked? Were you able to stay in charge because you called a friend or went for a walk? How do you think you could develop new skills to help you handle this problem more confidently in the future?

As fast as you can, write down all the ways you can think of to solve the problem. One winner had trouble resisting food at parties, particularly when standing beside a table of delectable hors d'oeuvres. That's when her confidence in her ability to control her eating dipped to its lowest ebb. Here's the list she drew up before attending her next office party.

- Don't stand by the hors d'oeuvres table.
- Strike up conversations with interesting people who are as far from the food table as possible.
- Chat about the latest news or gossip, not about how good the food is.
- Get one glass of white wine (or Evian water) and sip it slowly.
- Laugh a lot and enjoy the music.
- Keep yourself from feeling deprived by filling one small plate with just one or two bites of each food you'd like to sample. Savor each bite.
- Watch your social anxieties. When you feel shy and sense your anxiety mounting, take a time-out. Go to the ladies' room to brush your hair, or step outside on the veranda, patio, or porch for a few minutes.
- Look for friends who make you feel comfortable, and talk mostly to them.
- Watch out for competitive insults from certain coworkers (you know who). If you feel hurt, just raise your eyebrows archly and walk away. Do *not* walk toward the hors d'oeuvres table.

Armed with this self-designed list (very important), which she kept in her pocket for quick reference, she found it much easier to resist overeating at the party and was able to build her confidence in her ability to keep losing weight.

3. TROUBLESHOOT YOUR SOLUTIONS

Suppose your plan doesn't work. Then you need to ask why. Did anything at all work, even just a little? If so, which strategies worked best? What unexpected problems cropped up? How could you get around those obstacles and do better next time? Becoming the scientist of your own body involves testing out theories, seeing where they went wrong, then calmly trying again.

What if you zero in on one particularly tough problem area and find yourself thinking, "There's *no way* I can resist eating in that situation. It's hopeless"? Don't despair. That's just your cortisol talking. You've given up on yourself—temporarily. But you can bolster your confidence again.

How? Get your effort hormones flowing again by focusing on your searching behavior. If you truly have no clue how you might solve this particular problem, try talking it over with a diet buddy or other good friend. Or go on the Internet, tap into a dieters' newsgroup, and see how other women have solved similar problems.

Still no luck? Then take a break for a while. Relax by enjoying a task that will lower the no-confidence cortisol in your system. Meditate for twenty minutes. Listen to peaceful music. Go buy a book of Cathy cartoons and laugh at all *her* eating problems. Take a calm, energizing walk. Once you feel more positive, go back to your troubleshooting list. The goal isn't to find immediate answers. The goal is to keep trying and generating new ideas. Remember, you can't make a mistake. There is no trial and error, only trial and learning. Once you've found a solution that *didn't* work, you're in a better position to find one that will.

4. ASK, "WHERE'S THE THREAT?"

When you feel stress mounting, take five deep breaths (see "Relaxation Quickie: The Breath Focus" on page 109), then check out your feelings. Ask, "How am I feeling right now? What's going on here?" And, most important, "Where's the *threat?*" Daily Hassles Fat almost always involves some threat you fear you can't handle. When you analyze the situation more closely, you'll often realize you have far more resources than you originally thought.

Tracey, twenty-nine, a copywriter with a large Chicago advertising agency, felt constantly hassled at work. As a result, she was so distressed when she got home at night she couldn't stop snacking. Even if she ate a satisfying dinner with dessert, within an hour she would be looking for something sweet and fattening to nibble on to lift her spirits. When she began taking mental notes during the day, she realized the bulk of her hassles came from two coworkers who occupied large chunks of her time. They would come into her office, sit on her couch, complain about their jobs—and keep her from getting her work done. This happened maybe four, even five days a week, usually between 2 and 4 P.M. As a result, she was always stressed-out and pressed for time. Often she even had to work all weekend to keep from missing a deadline.

When she asked "Where's the threat?" she realized her only fear was that she'd alienate these two complainers. Would this get her fired? No. In fact, it might save her job. Tracey began closing her office door every afternoon and letting everyone know that a closed door meant she should *not* be disturbed. At last able to get on top of her work, she found it much easier to relax and stop nibbling at night. In six months, she lost 43 pounds. (Eventually, one of the whiners quit; the other got fired.)

5. TURN YOUR INNER CRITIC INTO A CHEERLEADER

When we're stressed, we almost always look for those problems *outside* ourselves to see what stirred us up. But stress—and Daily Hassles Fat—also springs from *internal* stressors. Superconfidence is an inside job; and so is low confidence. Daily Hassles Fat often goes hand in hand with an inner critic who makes comments like "Dwelling on what you've done right only makes you a braggart (or complacent)," "I've gotten where I am by never accepting less than perfection," and "I'm my own worst critic." We repeat these lessons with pride, as if we have to jump the gun and criticize ourselves *first* before anyone else does. Those of us who as kids were taught never to "boast in public" often learned the lesson so well we now fail to give ourselves *inner* pep talks.

Winners who beat Daily Hassles Fat beat externally generated stress by learning to say no to unreasonable demands. But they also beat *internally* generated stress by giving themselves mental applause and self-praise. Rather than being their own worst critic, they become their own best cheerleaders. This attitude affects more than their weight: it pervades their whole lives. At Trent University in Ontario, Canada, women who *continued* to lose weight on their own after a weight-control program ended were compared with those who quickly began to backslide without expert support. The women who took charge often agreed with statements like these:

> "When I realize I'll be unavoidably late for an important meeting, I tell myself to keep calm." (Likewise, when winners temporarily blow their diets, they tell themselves to calm down.)
> "When I'm short on money, I decide to record all my expenses in order to budget more carefully in the future." (Similarly, when they start regaining weight, winners decide to record

their problems in a journal in order to avoid those same mistakes in the future.)

"I prefer to finish a job that I have to do before I start doing things I really like to do." (Ask yourself this: Would you rather finish a job you've been working on diligently for over a year or start fresh on an exciting new project? Winners love the joy of a good finish.)

"When I succeed at small things, I become encouraged to go on." (Likewise, winners build on small wins. Just losing a few pounds encourages them to move on; they don't have to lose 50 pounds in a month to feel better.)

"The way I achieve my goals is by rewarding myself every step along the way." (Likewise, winners often give themselves little nonedible "rewards"—like a day off, a new book, or a massage—for losing as little as 2 pounds in a week.)

As one woman turned off her mental critic and learned to give herself mental applause, she discovered she was much less apt to stress-eat *because she had much less stress*. She's kept off 32 pounds of Daily Hassles Fat for five years.

6. MIX HASSLES WITH "BREATHERS"

Throughout the day, notice when your stress levels start to mount and take tiny steps *at the time* to soothe yourself before your cortisol climbs. "If a client calls in a foul mood and reads me the riot act, I try not to react emotionally," says Jane, a public-relations consultant. "But I take a quick emotional check. If I find I *am* reacting (for me, the clues are that my breathing has gotten more shallow and my jaw tightens), then I release the tension right then and there by taking a few deep, soothing breaths and consciously relaxing my jaw. After every ninety minutes or so, I'll get up from my desk, stretch, and take a quick walk down the hall. Or maybe I'll just switch gears. If I've been working nonstop on a presentation for two hours and feel myself tensing up, I'll stop for twenty minutes and make a few phone calls." Since she began taking "de-stress breaks" every two hours or so, she notes, "It's been much easier for me to cut back on my eating when I've gained two or three pounds." She also no longer has headaches.

As Jane's experience suggests, many winners view small stress-related symptoms—a stiff neck, aching back, or throbbing head—as secret messages from their unconscious telling them they're living too much according to others' rules instead of their own. During their breaks they "turn off" external pressures and tune back into their own rhythms, often by focusing on their breathing (see below).

Judith, a busy mother of three, pencils in pleasures on her to-do list. Sandwiched between chores like "take Bobbie to soccer practice" and "go to the cleaners," she jots items that feed her deeper needs, like "daydream for twenty minutes," "go to an 11 A.M. showing of that new romantic movie," and "sit outside in the sun and feel at one with the world." She notes, "I've learned that having free time for myself really helps reduce my stress eating, so I now work 'free' time right into my schedule." By filling her days with little rewards to balance the hassles, she has lost 86 pounds.

Relaxation Quickie: The Breath Focus

Some of us are so stressed we can hardly breathe. Our breath is restricted, shallow, nervous, and tight. Weight-control winners frequently become masters of deep breathing because it's such a simple way to de-stress and relax the stomach (where overweight women often carry their tension). To learn to breathe "correctly" (taking deep, relaxing breaths as opposed to shallow stress-ridden ones), inhale from the belly, not the chest.

Put one hand on your abdomen, the other on your chest. Then breathe slowly and deeply through your nose. When you're breathing to beat stress, your abdomen will expand like a balloon. As you exhale through your mouth with a long, slow, deep sigh, let your abdomen deflate. Imagine that the air you breathe in carries with it a sense of calm and peace, while the air going out carries away all tension and anxiety. Anytime you're stuck in traffic or caught in a long checkout line, take a huge, cleansing breath. Hold it for four seconds, then exhale very slowly. Feel the tension drain from your body. Focus especially on relaxing your stomach.

7. Stop Watching the News

In one *British Journal of Psychology* study, people who watched a mere fourteen minutes of negative news became sadder, more anxious, and more likely to "catastrophize" their own personal worries. Four years ago (shortly before she permanently lost 42 pounds), Tara reduced her daily hassles immensely when she stopped watching negative news on TV. She just went cold turkey. "All those rapes, murders, fires, floods, and wars just made me feel depressed and helpless [cortisol reactions] because I empathized with all those poor people but couldn't do a damned thing about their problems. I'd sit there night after night, watching the news, feeling helpless, angry, and out of control. Then I'd raid the refrigerator."

If you haven't already done it, you might also want to avoid violent movies. Even *fantasizing* about distressing problems beyond your control can heighten cortisol levels and lead to a spare tire. In one Italian study, healthy young women were shown forty-five minutes of violent scenes from one movie and a forty-five minute sequence of flowers, colors, and birds from Disney's *Fantasia*. While watching the violence, the women's minds and bodies went on red alert. Their heart rates and systolic blood pressure rose, and their no-confidence cortisol levels soared. *Fantasia* didn't produce this stress reaction. What's more, a Yale study found that under circumstances when cortisol rises, women eat more fattening foods. (Maybe that's why we feel "compelled" to scarf so much buttered popcorn while watching those gory movies.)

Daily Hassles Fat Quickie

To nurture her needs in nonfattening ways, one Connecticut winner keeps a list on her refrigerator door of the "21 Things I Love Most to Do That Don't Involve Food." Among them: drive through the countryside, pet the cat, go browse through the bookshop, build a fireplace fire and watch the flickering flames, read haiku poetry, arrange flowers, practice my birdcalls, listen to music, and write in my journal. She not only has a beautiful life, but she's kept off 76 pounds for three years.

8. LET YOURSELF BE NEEDY

In a University of Kansas study, 80 percent of women with only a few pounds to lose were most likely to eat at times when they felt "soft" and "gentle." Why? Possibly because many strong, independent women nowadays are trying to succeed in business by keeping our softer side under wraps. Struggling to maintain control when we feel gentle or "weak," we panic and spin completely *out* of control.

The answer: let your needy side show. Emotionally healthy winners aren't either/or types. Able to express many sides of their natures, they're comfortable being both strong *and* weak, tough *and* tender, independent *and* needy, in charge *and* able to let others take charge. Embodying many "selves" and able to flow easily from one state to another, they rarely bump into a "threatening" mood that triggers stress.

When Susan, a $200,000-a-year financial adviser, arrives home from the office, she's delighted to stop being in charge. "When my husband asks, 'What do you want to do tonight?' I'll often reply, 'Whatever you want, dear.' It's a relief to float free and let someone else make the decisions for a change." Asked how she can relinquish her hard-won power so easily to "please a man," she just laughs and replies, "I'm doing this to please *me*, to give myself time to unwind. Besides, our marriage isn't about power, it's about love. If I sound 'unliberated,' God help me, so be it. Frankly, I feel superliberated. Six years ago, I learned to go with the flow, and it helped me shed 50 pounds!"

When trying to strike a similar balance in your own life, think *rhythm*. At one point in your day, you may be the assertive, competitive dynamo. At another point, the independence fades, the softness flows in, and you're ready to let go and feel gentle. Poet Walt Whitman wrote, "Do I contradict myself? Very well, then I contradict myself. (I am large, I contain multitudes.)" It may take awhile to work out a rhythmic balance that feels right to you. But once you come to respect the independent and needy parts of your nature, you'll find that you can draw strength from both—and you'll feel less need to relieve stress with food.

9. BREAK YOUR BAD HABITS

Unfortunately, when we try to cope with our daily hassles, we often adopt habits that only make matters worse. Bad habits that can lead to Daily Hassles Fat include smoking, taking too many tranquilizers, drinking too much alcohol, and, possibly, consuming high amounts of caffeine.

Cigarette smokers, even thin ones, have more unhealthy visceral fat than nonsmokers. It's tucked deep inside the abdomen around vital organs, where you can't necessarily see it. But visible or not, it's still doing its metabolic damage. You have to remember, we're talking about *billions* of microscopic fat cells here. A smoker can look thin and still have billions of visceral fat cells busily spewing out free fatty acids and other damaging chemicals inside her body. So if you haven't already kicked the habit yet, this may be another reason to try.

Alcohol can also add to your visceral fat and make weight loss a lot harder. When you drink alcohol, your body has no place to store it. It has no alcohol-storage compartments. So the alcohol gets burned first, and any food you just ate gets stored until the alcohol is all gone. A Swiss study reported in the *New England Journal of Medicine* found if you're on a 1,250-calorie diet and get a mere 250 of those calories from beer, liquor, or wine, the alcohol can slow down your metabolism by 36 percent. Calories don't automatically lead to unhealthy stress fat. But calories *plus alcohol* may do so. So when you're trying to lose weight, you may want to abstain.

What about coffees, cola, and tea? Does caffeine make you fat? Theoretically it shouldn't. In a study done at King's College, University of London, a single cup of coffee increased previously overweight women's metabolic rates by 3 to 4 percent over the next 150 minutes. So caffeine might help you lose weight, or perhaps maintain your losses.

But here's the rub. Caffeine can also cause your body to release cortisol, so you may feel compelled to eat more fat than you otherwise would. If you're struggling with Night-Eating Syndrome, caffeine could also keep you awake. Also, some evidence suggests caffeine coupled with stress may raise your blood pressure, if you have a family history of hypertension. So while caffeine may cause most people no problems, there may be a "caffeine-sensitive" subgroup it does hurt.

Because the most popular caffeinated drinks—coffee, tea, and diet sodas—contain no calories, they're often considered a dieter's friend, something you can drink to your heart's content. But if you're drinking a lot of caffeine, you might ask yourself this: Could all this caffeine be contributing to my weight in some way? Only you can decide, because only you know your own body. But it's something to think about. Just check it out. You might want to give up coffee for a month and see if or how it affects your weight. You may also sleep better, another important factor for preventing weight gain. See Chapter 15, "Losing Night-Eating Fat," for more about this and for ways to get a slimming night's sleep.

10. TAKE "MINI-VACATIONS"

In place of bad habits that only thicken your waistline, try to carve out quiet time—anywhere from a few minutes to an hour a day—to re-center yourself. Valerie, a California mother of two, has kept 22 pounds off for three years by taking what she calls a "meditation walk" each afternoon. "I just put the kids in a stroller and walk through a neighborhood park, looking at the roses, listening to the mockingbirds, and noticing the beauty of nature."

As often as she can on her lunch hours, Kimberly, a criminal attorney who lost 52 pounds, retreats to a public library near her office to read trashy romance novels. "It's my way of telling myself to lighten up."

Amanda, an air-traffic controller, takes twenty minutes to unwind every day when she gets home from work. She simply goes into her favorite room (a combination plant room and study), locks the door, and daydreams she's at the beach. "I can see the waves spraying against the rocks, hear the seagulls crying, and even taste the salty air," she says. "At first my three kids kept trying to interrupt, but I gently reminded them they could talk to their father until I came out. Now they respect my private time. Just twenty minutes a day. It may not sound like much. But for me, it's a lifesaver." After this "mini-vacation," she can prepare and eat dinner calmly without stuffing herself.

CHAPTER 10

Losing Depression Fat

The eternal stars shine out as soon as it is dark enough.

—*Thomas Carlyle*

Shortly after her third miscarriage, Anna's weight began spiraling out of control. Once a svelte 123 pounds, she ballooned up to 162 in less than a year. "I was thirty-four and beginning to fear I'd never have children," she recalls. "I couldn't understand why I was getting so fat because I really *didn't* eat that much—or at least I didn't think I did."

Although Anna didn't know it, depression leads to extremely high cortisol levels. In fact, another name for depression is "hypercortisolism" (*hyper* means "high"). This means when you're depressed, you can gain weight, even when you *don't* overeat. Some women with extreme cases of Depression Fat have been overloaded with cortisol for so long they resemble battle-fatigue victims. They've succumbed to a full-blown case of the Civilization Syndrome: *distress without effort.*

If you were among this sadly overwhelmed group, you wouldn't be reading this page. The fact that you're here confirms you're still making an effort, still searching for answers. Fortunately, help is at hand.

If depression has tormented you for months or years, seeking out a competent, supportive therapist can be an empowering step toward tracking down your solutions. But there's another kind of help that doesn't require leaving your house. Nor does it cost you a dime. It's the help from your very own "therapist within."

Often, the hardest part about relying on your inner therapist is trusting that even when you're deeply troubled, you still contain a font of hidden wisdom you can draw on for solutions. Trust yourself, and believe it. Though psychoanalyst Carl Jung was the first to describe "the wisdom of the unconscious," it's now widely recognized and has even been documented in peer-reviewed journals.

Is This Your Problem?

1. Do you often feel depressed and unable to enjoy life for most of the day nearly every day?
2. When you're feeling blue, do you try to boost your mood with food?
3. Have you experienced a significant weight gain, especially around the midsection?
4. Do you have trouble sleeping or, conversely, do you sleep too much?
5. Do you feel constantly agitated or barely able to drag yourself through your day?
6. Do you often feel guilty?
7. Do you have trouble making a decision, thinking, or concentrating?
8. Do you have recurring thoughts of death and even thoughts of suicide?

If you answered yes to most of these questions (especially 1 through 3), you're probably struggling with Depression Fat. If you've had at least five of these symptoms for more than two weeks, you may also have a major depression that needs to be treated.

In one classic study reported in the *British Medical Journal*, researchers tracked down forty-nine out of seventy-six patients who—due to overcrowding at one psychiatric clinic—had been wait-listed but never received treatment: 65 percent had either improved or recovered. (Therapists call such self-healings "spontaneous remissions.") That's not to say these people cured themselves with no help at all. They may have received helpful counsel from family and friends. But, clearly, you contain more self-healing power than you might imagine.

We seldom recognize depression as a stress reaction. We may think it's a personal "flaw." But, in fact, Depression Fat is a high-cortisol reaction; it means you're so overwhelmed by stress you've practically come to a halt. We've all heard that angry people are more prone to heart disease. What's less well known is that depression—and Depression Fat—may be equally hard on your heart. In an investigation by researchers at Duke University Medical Center, Danish women and men whose psychological tests revealed low self-esteem, lack of motivation, concentration problems, and despair were 70 percent more likely to have a heart attack and 60 percent more likely to die over the next ten years than people who felt happier.

If you're overweight and depressed—and you also eat to assuage your depression (that's how you cope)—you have two interconnected problems: the overeating and the depression. The best way to handle these problems, winners report, is to tackle them separately. First, you need to develop the ability to stop eating when you're depressed (many tips in Chapters 9 and 13 should help you with this). Second, you need to find ways to bolster your moods, so you'll be less depressed (and therefore less likely to store fat in your unhealthy visceral zone). These lessons from winners will help you do both:

1.Use Solutions You've Already Found

Remember, nothing *always* happens. Although you may think you feel sad all the time, you undoubtedly have bright spots in your day or week when you feel better than usual. On a scale from 0 to 10 (from 0 being so depressed you can't get out of bed to 10 being euphoric), where are you right now? If you're at a 3, great! You're higher than a lot of people. What do you think you could do to get up to a 4?

Think back to the last time you had a reasonably good day, one on which you didn't have to eat to boost your spirits. What made that day different? What did you do on your "reasonably good day" that you might try again to create other good days? Did you eat more *regularly* than usual or have breakfast for a change? (Depression often springs from dieting too much, especially meal skipping.)

Did you call a friend, listen to music, read a good book, get a massage, or go for a walk?

Notice those mood lifters that work; do more of them. Notice those experiments that fall flat; do something else.

2. Go with Your Body's Flow

Your moods and energy naturally rise and fall throughout the day. "It's extremely important to pay attention to these energy cycles," says Robert Thayer, a psychology professor at California State University, Long Beach, and author of *The Origin of Everyday Moods*. Ignoring them is one thing that leads to stress, depression—and overeating.

You may even want to keep a "mood diary" to see how your moods change from day to day or even hour to hour. It's a great way to gain self-insight. Once you recognize that your moods have a rhythmic pattern, you'll be less likely to conclude "it's the end of the world" whenever you've merely hit a predictable low.

Mood patterns vary among individuals. But for most of us, energy (and positive feelings) peak between 11 A.M. and 1 P.M. That's the time to notice how good you feel, to relish your "natural high." When your energy is at its lowest—around 4 P.M. and from 9 P.M. to 11 P.M.—try to take it easy. Phone a friend, practice yoga, go to the flower shop, hum a little song, write a silly poem, or take a hot bath. These are definitely *not* moments to dwell on your problems or pick a fight with your spouse. If you do, you'll pig out on pizza for sure.

3. Use Active Mood Boosters

When we're feeling blue, many of us use passive mood boosters. We drink coffee, watch TV, have a cocktail, smoke a cigarette, or eat a candy bar in an attempt to feel better. As you now know, these strategies often release cortisol. They may give you a temporary lift. But an hour or so later, they'll backfire, and you'll feel even worse.

The very best ways to lift a bad mood involve some kind of *effort*. It seems to go against all logic, but when you're too tired, sad, or lethargic to do something positive—to take a brisk ten-minute walk, lift weights, dance, or organize your desk—that's exactly what you need to do. In a small study at Duke University involving depressed people over age fifty, short but strenuous workouts—as little as eight minutes long—temporarily but dramatically reduced depressive symptoms. After brief workouts, the over-fifties reported an 82 percent reduction in feelings of depression, tension, anger, confusion, and fatigue. No matter how depressed they'd been beforehand, they felt more vigorous and energetic after they'd exercised. The real power of exercise when you're battling Depression Fat may not be the number of calories it burns (which can be fairly insignificant), but the depression it relieves. After a brisk walk, you may feel energized—and happier—for hours.

4. FIND YOUR HIDDEN OPTIMIST

We're often taught that the world is divided into two types of people: pessimists (who frequently display *distress without effort*) and optimists (who more often exhibit *effort without distress*). Such black-and-white thinking distorts reality. In fact, we all have both optimistic and pessimistic tendencies. When you're struggling with Depression Fat, the pessimistic part of you has simply gotten the upper hand. Temporarily.

Fortunately, we can all *learn* to be more hopeful. We craft our own minds to embrace hope or despair. How optimistic you stay day after day, how eagerly you continue to make an effort, depends largely on what University of Pennsylvania psychologist Martin E. P. Seligman calls your *explanatory style* (how you explain the misfortunes that come your way).

Weight-loss winners seldom feel helpless and depressed for long. They bounce quickly back from defeat. We've already seen one way they do it: they keep searching for answers. They also stay optimistic. How? Seligman, who has devoted his life to answering this question, believes optimism is learned in three ways. Develop these three attitudes, and you'll help the optimist within you resurface.

First, learn to see "good" events and their causes as *permanent*. When an optimist succeeds at turning down a piece of cheesecake at her sister's house, she'll tend to declare: "I'm a superconfident winner. I always achieve what I set out to do. Another victory for me." The pessimist within, who sees "good" events as temporary, may waffle: "Well, I did okay that time, but it was only once, and I was probably just lucky."

Conversely, when "bad" events happen, your inner optimist views the causes as *temporary:* When she eats a piece of cheesecake the size of a Frisbee, she explains: "I was exhausted (I learned a valuable lesson)"; or "Diets just don't work when I go to my sister's house for dinner (I need to figure out why)." The inner pessimist says, "I'm all washed up" and "Diets never work, anyway. Screw it."

Second, view your success as *pervasive.* When you succeed in one area of your life, the optimist within uses this victory as a super-confident springboard to help you achieve your next goal. Example: When you did well on a tough project at work, your inner optimist cheers, "Wow, I did really well on that project. I can learn anything. With enough work, I can be a weight-loss winner, too." The pessimist says, "Whew! That project was a real bear. I'm glad I dodged that bullet. Never again!"

Third, *personalize* and *internalize* the positive events in your life. Take credit for everything that goes right. "Of course I lost weight," the optimist in you beams. "I took charge and designed my own diet. I have inner strengths. I can solve any problem that crops up." The glowering pessimist *externalizes* your success: "I only lost weight because of that Sue Browder. She's my guru. I could never have done it on my own."

Hold on here, the skeptic in you may be thinking. All this positive thinking sounds great, but doesn't depression have a strong hereditary component? You're right, it does. Some people do inherit a genetic *susceptibility* toward depression, but biology is not destiny. It's still activated by the choices we make. As you now know, mind/body disorders aren't *either* genetic *or* environmental. They're *both.* So even if you have inherited a tendency toward depression, you can still bring out your hidden optimist with a little positive thinking. You can take charge of your thoughts. When you do, you'll be amazed how much your depression will lift.

Five Ways to Beat "Winter Fat"

One subtype of depression fat is Winter Fat, thought to be caused by too little sunlight and disrupted circadian rhythms. Scientists have dubbed this well-publicized condition seasonal affective disorder, or SAD.

When depressed or discouraged, 57 percent of female SAD sufferers eat sweets (particularly chocolate, cakes, and pastries), 18 percent head for starchy foods like potatoes, 21 percent medicate their moods with caffeine, and 14 percent drink alcohol. An estimated 17 percent of people in the United States may struggle with Winter Fat at some point in their lives.

To find relief:

1. Get more sunlight. Spending time outside, even on a cloudy day, exposes you to more of the sun's rays than you'll get indoors. An early morning or lunchtime walk in the sunshine—without sunglasses—is ideal.
2. Try an artificial light box. About 75 percent of SAD sufferers get fast relief from special light boxes, which are five to twenty times brighter than the lighting typically found in most homes.
3. Boost your mood with exercise. If they can't get outside, winners ride stationary bikes, dance to their favorite music, and jump rope. It all helps.
4. Don't fight your cravings. Swiss scientists recently found that SAD sufferers who ate more than one portion of sweets during the afternoon or evening usually responded to light treatment. Once they got more light, their cravings usually diminished.
5. See a doctor for serious SAD symptoms. Fatigue coupled with increased appetite can also signal low blood sugar or a thyroid disorder (in which case you may have Lazy Thyroid Fat).

5. Ask, "What Have I Lost?"

Whereas Daily Hassles Fat usually springs from some *threat*, Depression Fat typically springs from a *loss*. Any loss—from having your car stolen to a hypothetical loss like worrying that you'll get cancer—can propel you toward the fridge. But so can subtler losses, such as unresolved grief over your mother's death twenty years ago, the fact you've "lost" a talent you no longer use, or a "loss of face" from looking bad on the job.

To pinpoint the loss that's got you bogged down, sit quietly, do one of your deep-breathing exercises, and stop hating the fact you're depressed. (When we tell ourselves we "shouldn't" feel this way, we become *depressed about being depressed*, which of course only make matters worse.) Quiet your agitation. Do nothing. Calmly observe the stillness. Ask your depression, "Why are you here?"

Once you've pinpointed why you're so blue, it's important to ask a second question: What can I *gain* from this insight? What meaning can you find in this loss? How can you use this setback, loneliness, or grief to grow stronger? In our noisy world, being forced to withdraw silently into yourself may be a gift in disguise. You suddenly have time to hear that "still, small voice within." What is she trying to tell you?

Some winners find what they once viewed as a "bad" depressive episode turned out to be the prelude to a period of immense creativity. It's almost as if they had to fall apart before they could put themselves back together again in new, more authentic ways. Laurel, a winner from Portland, Oregon, says: "I'd had some low-level depression for years, but it got really bad when I hit forty. I thought, 'What am I doing with my life?' It all felt so empty." Once Laurel began accepting her depression as a *teacher* (not as a curse), she began using it as a springboard to self-insight. "As I spent time contemplating my life, I realized I'd always been creative and spontaneous, so why was I working as an accountant (which I hated)? I was completely off my path, and some part of me knew it." Laurel went back to school, got a degree in education, and now teaches art and writing to gifted children. As her vitality blossomed, almost as a side effect, she shed 35 pounds.

Are such postdepression transformations rare? No. In fact, they may be quite common. Carl Jung, who studied hundreds of educated people during his lifetime, observed that of those over age thirty-five who came to him with "psychic sufferings" like mental depression, *not one* person recovered without finding some spiritual answers. Losses that lead to the darkness can also lead back to the light.

Is St. John's Wort for You?

Many women are reluctant to take "hard-core" antidepressant SSRI drugs like Zoloft or Paxil or the tricyclics like amitriptyline or imipramine, for fear they'll lead to weight gain. Is the herb St. John's wort an alternative if you're only moderately depressed? Maybe so.

A randomized, double-blind, controlled study done in Germany and published in an international peer-reviewed pharmacology journal compared St. John's wort with Prozac for treatment of mild to moderate depression. There was one main difference: St. John's wort was safer. Significant side effects were reported by 23 percent of people taking Prozac versus only 8 percent on St. John's wort. The most common effects of Prozac included agitation (8 percent), gastrointestinal disturbances (6 percent), retching and dizziness (4 percent each). The only significant side effects of St. John's wort were gastrointestinal disturbances, reported by 5 percent of patients.

St. John's wort may also relieve the Depression Fat associated with menopause and seasonal affective disorder. In a *British Medical Journal* study, the standard dose of St. John's wort (which proved just as effective as imipramine) was 350 milligrams three times a day. Herbs are not FDA-regulated in the United States, however. So you need to be careful about the source of any herbs you use. Also, be sure to let your health provider know what you're doing.

6. Be Aware of Gaslighting

Not *all* depression springs from a spiritual crisis. Many negative emotions have their root in unhappy interaction with other people. If your husband, "friends," or relatives continually put you down in some way, you may wind up confused, depressed, and fat—but not quite know why.

In the classic film *Gaslight*, the character played by Charles Boyer constantly turned the lights up and down and played other devious tricks to chip away at the self-esteem of his young bride (Ingrid Bergman) and make her think she was going crazy. A similar kind of depression-promoting behavior often goes on in many relationships. George Bach and Peter Wyden, authors of *The Intimate Enemy*, have called it "gaslighting."

If you grew up in a verbally abusive home, you may be especially vulnerable to this type of disrespect. You may have a hard time recognizing it. Disparaging comments like "You're just too sensitive,"

"You're always making a big deal out of nothing," and "You can't take a joke" or direct squelches like "Who asked you?" or "Nobody asked your opinion" can leave you feeling depressed and lonely for legitimate reasons. Unless you can validate your feelings (I *feel* put down, I *am* being put down; I *feel* hurt, I *am* being hurt), you may wind up heading for the kitchen to assuage your pain and find "love" in the form of food.

In her book *The Verbally Abusive Relationship*, communications expert Patricia Evans lists many categories of verbal abuse, including:

Discounting: "You always take things wrong," "You're not happy unless you're complaining," "You have no sense of humor."

Insults disguised as jokes: "You couldn't find your head if it wasn't glued on," "What else can you expect from a woman?"

Blocking and diverting: "You heard me; I shouldn't have to repeat myself," "Just drop it," "Where did you get a dumb idea like that?"

Accusing and blaming: "Now you've made me angry again," "It's all your fault," "I've had it with your attacks/bitching/complaining," "You're always looking for trouble."

Denial: "I never said that," "There's nothing wrong, you're just PMSing," "I don't know where you got that," "You're making that up."

If these conversations sound like a tape recording of your home life, Depression Fat may very well be the way you're attempting to cope with an extremely unhappy and difficult situation. Until you can recognize verbal abuse for what it is and either find a way to escape or learn how to ask for change calmly (realizing you deserve to be treated with respect), Depression Fat may provide self-protection and even some level of safety. This is not to say you're doing anything "wrong." You're currently coping in the best way you know how with problems you can solve only in your own way. But know this: you *do* have the inner strength to solve them.

If and when you're ready for change, Evans's excellent book *The Verbally Abusive Relationship* is a good place to begin gaining insight. Also start thinking of ways you can create a support network of friends and relatives who can help. (In an emergency, see "When

Fat Signals Danger . . ." on page 92.) Some overweight women feel both depressed *and* angry, a condition termed "agitated depression." If your sadness alternates with anger attacks, Chapter 12, "Losing Anger Fat," should help.

CHAPTER 11

Losing Lazy Thyroid Fat

Of all the sly, subtle problems that can affect physical or mental health, none is more common than thyroid gland disturbance.

—*Broda O. Barnes, M.D.*

In her twenties, Laurie was an administrative assistant who survived on junk food and ate whatever she pleased. If she gained 5 pounds, no problem. She could lose them in a week just by cutting back on the fries. Suddenly, in her mid-thirties, however, her stress levels began skyrocketing, and so did her weight. "I was attending college at night, studying for my M.B.A., while working a full-time job and keeping in touch with my mother, who was dying from cancer. As a result, I was smoking two packs of cigarettes a day, eating poorly, pumping myself up with caffeine, and sleeping as little as four hours a night. In two years, my dress size shot up from a six to an eighteen!"

Laurie stopped smoking at her doctor's insistence, but only gained only another 10 pounds. "I also often felt cold, my eyes were all dry and puffy, and I had bruises that just wouldn't heal. Once I jammed my thumb really hard, and three months later, it was still black and blue. I had no idea all these bizarre symptoms, including my weight, were *connected*."

Eventually, Laurie could barely drag herself out of bed, and her doctor ordered blood tests. The diagnosis: an underactive thyroid. Laurie is one of the estimated thirteen million people (mostly women) in the United States who either have Lazy Thyroid Fat or may soon develop it. Medically known as hypothyroidism, this disorder goes undiagnosed so frequently it's been called "the disease doctors often ignore."

The thyroid is a butterfly-shaped gland in your throat at the base of your Adam's apple. It produces two hormones (T-4 and T-3) that influence every cell, tissue, and organ in your body, including brain cells. This gland also controls your metabolism. When it gets "lazy" or sluggish, your metabolism plummets and the weight piles on.

Hypothyroidism comes from *hypo*, meaning "low." Women with the opposite condition (*hyper*thyroidism, from *hyper* for "high") develop wolfish appetites and become rail thin, despite ravenous eating.

As many as one in ten overweight women may suffer from hypothyroidism, and the risk increases with each decade after age thirty-four. Women are five times more likely to develop Lazy Thyroid Fat than men. No one knows why. But the wide hormonal swings that accompany pregnancy may play a role. About half the women with this condition have no idea what's wrong with them.

Anita, who edits a newsletter on at-home-businesses, developed Lazy Thyroid Fat in a sudden spurt. Since she was already taking medication for her thyroid (she'd had a thyroid condition since her teens), she didn't connect her rapid weight gain to the change one doctor had made in her prescription. She knew only that her weight had skyrocketed from 114 to 308 pounds in less than six months. Struggling to lose even so little as half a pound, she went from doctor to doctor. Their constant refrain: eat less, exercise more. Convinced by now that her weight was completely her fault, she redoubled her efforts. Once she fasted on water only for nearly a month—and gained three pounds. "On one hand, I knew the doctors were missing something. Yet another part of me kept saying I couldn't trust my own feelings and I must be crazy. Many people in my life have tried to tell me what's going on in my body isn't real. I was embarrassed that I felt so rotten."

Anita found an astute gynecologist who told her she had a thyroid problem. "When he said it was impossible for me to lose weight until I got my hormones back in balance, I felt almost euphoric. At last! Someone finally believed me and understood that it wasn't my fault."

As she left the doctor's office and went home, she cried off and on for several hours with relief. Once she got back on the right medication for *her* (the one she'd originally been taking), Anita lost 60 pounds in three months—with no change in her eating habits. At last report, she'd lost 145 pounds and was still dropping. It had taken her seven long years, but she'd finally found her solution. Now *that's* superconfident persistence.

Unfortunately, if left untreated, hypothyroidism can do more than just make you fat. As your thyroid hormones fall, your risk of heart disease rises. This especially unhealthy way to be fat definitely needs to be diagnosed and treated.

Is This Your Problem?

Are you always tired or run-down?

Do you feel cold and need to wear a sweater when others feel warm?

Do you have dry, scaly skin, a puffy face and eyes, or dry, brittle nails and hair?

Do you feel foggy or have trouble concentrating and remembering things?

Do you have heavy periods or irregular menstrual cycles? Infertility problems?

Is your cholesterol high—even a little?

Do you sometimes have "pins and needles" sensations in your fingers and toes?

Do you frequently feel depressed or blue?

Do you have joint and muscle pains?

Do you have a family history of thyroid problems or insulin-dependent diabetes?

Do you have white skin spots?

If you answered yes to any of these questions, a Lazy Thyroid may be at the root of your problems, and you need to get tested.

How to Tell If You Have It

Aside from weight gain, common symptoms of hypothyroidism include fatigue, cold intolerance, dry itchy skin, muscle cramps, a puffy face, brittle hair, difficulty concentrating, and other symptoms listed on page 127. Unfortunately, such symptoms are so vague and general, they're often attributed to stress, menopause, depression, or even just ordinary aging. It's also common for doctors to get sidetracked by a single symptom (severe headaches or heavy periods, for example) and concentrate on treating that symptom rather than getting to the root of the problem. Some women with lazy thyroids even wind up having unnecessary hysterectomies, which may only make matters worse. (See "Another Way Your Doctor Can Make You Fat"on page 194.)

How can you tell if you have Lazy Thyroid Fat? The best way is to get your thyroid tested by a doctor. But here's a simple, home self-test you can try tomorrow. Place an ordinary mercury thermometer on your nightstand before you go to sleep tonight. When you first awaken in the morning, tuck the thermometer into your armpit, and lie back down. Lie quietly for fifteen minutes. Then check your temperature and record it on a piece of paper. Do this for five consecutive days. If your temperature is below 97.6 every day, you may have Lazy Thyroid Fat and need to ask your doctor for a very sensitive (third generation) TSH test.

What's that? TSH is short for thyroid-stimulating hormone. When your thyroid gets sluggish, your pituitary gland tries to kick it back into gear by secreting more TSH. If the thyroid fails to respond, the pituitary secretes even more TSH. In other words, *high* levels of TSH in your blood indicate *low* thyroid function.

Every doctor knows how to do this simple test. But if you have the luxury of choosing your own doctor (not always possible in this HMO age), try to find a good clinician who will treat you as an equal partner in your own healing.

Once you're diagnosed, the usual treatment is a daily dose of the synthetic thyroid drug levothyroxine (lee-voh-thy-ROX-een), sold under the brand names Synthroid, Levothroid, Levosine, or Levo-T. It can be tricky to achieve exactly the right dose for you as a unique individual. It's best to start low and work up. That's why you need a caring, diligent doctor to carefully fine-tune your dosage until you begin feeling better and start losing weight.

If you're lucky, this treatment alone will restore your energy and resolve your weight problems. Just one caution: as Anita's

example illustrates well, once you've established a dose that's
ing, don't play around with it or switch medications (dif
brands can vary in their concentrations and even name brands like
Synthroid have had fluctuating-potency problems). Still, if all goes
well, in a few months you'll be thin.

Troubleshooting Your Treatment

Let's suppose that not everything goes smoothly. Let's say you're
now convinced from your symptoms and self-test that you do have
Lazy Thyroid Fat. Yet your doctor insists you don't. You're told
your TSH levels are "perfectly normal" and you just need to eat less
(a common occurrence). Should you scratch this possibility off your
list? Maybe, but not necessarily.

Before you do, ask how your doctor defines "normal." Even different testing labs have different ranges. What's known as "subclin-
ical hypothyroidism" (thyroid disease that hasn't yet progressed to
a full-blown disorder) can cause many women to gain weight, feel
lethargic, and experience other thyroid-related problems, even
when their TSH levels look fine.

So at exactly what readings *should* a lazy thyroid be treated?
That depends on who you ask. The American College of Physicians, a conservative, "evidence-based" medical organization, clas-
sifies 6 to 9 milli-international units per liter (mU/ls) as a "mildly
elevated" TSH reading. Above 10 is serious. Yet some patient activists insist they needed treatment even when their TSH readings
were under 4.5.

How low your TSH should be before your thyroid levels are
pronounced "normal" is also subject to debate. Many doctors classify any reading below 5 or 4.5 as normal. Yet some patients insist
they feel energetic and healthy only when their TSH levels are in
the "low normal" range, even as low as 1 or 2. Who's right?
Remember, you're the scientist of your own body. The right treatment is the one that feels best to you. If you feel lousy, especially if
your TSH is greater than 2 and you have a family history of thyroid disease, talk to your doctor about having a more sensitive
TRH (thyrotropin-releasing hormone) test, which can bring out
low thyroid levels that didn't show up on the TSH.

Is there any danger associated with taking medication you don't need? Absolutely, and that's another factor you need to consider. Too much thyroid hormone can lead to insomnia, nervousness, anxiety, hair loss, and possibly even heart disease and osteoporosis. When doing your own research, you have to remember there are huge profits to be made if drug companies can get millions of normal, healthy women on expensive, lifelong medications. It's important to apply a hefty dose of skepticism to anything you read on, say, the Internet about "patients' rights" to have the thyroid medications they "want." A Web site that looks like a legitimate patient-advocacy group may secretly be funded by a pharmaceutical company. Even some of the big medical research foundations have drug company backing and may be less reliable than they look. Your best bet, once again, is to find a good doctor you trust, preferably an endocrinologist who specializes in thyroid disorders. Ultimately, whether you need thyroid medication to slim down and deal with your other symptoms is a decision only you and your doctor can make together.

Here's a second thorny issue. Let's suppose you've been diagnosed with Lazy Thyroid Fat, and you're taking medication, but it's not working. You're still feeling low on energy, and you're still fat. Then you hear someone raving about the wonders of a "natural" thyroid drug. Is that your answer?

Good question. Let's explore it a minute. Most synthetic thyroid drugs on the market, at least at this writing, contain only one hormone: T-4, or thyroxine. Yet your thyroid actually makes *two* hormones: T-4 and T-3, or triiodothyronine. So why not replace them both? There's a simple explanation: T-4 converts to T-3 in your blood. So by taking just one hormone, you *are* getting them both. That's the short answer.

Now here's one that's a little longer. For fifty years, when the only available medication was the "natural" kind made from desiccated (dried and powdered) pig thyroid, both hormones *were* replaced. Unfortunately, that medication (still available and called Armour) led to heart problems in some people. When safer synthetics came on the market, Armour became obsolete, and most conventional doctors no longer prescribe it. Yet a few new mavericks and old-timers still believe the T-4/T-3 treatment is better, especially for women like Anita who have severe problems. What's more, recent evidence suggests they could be right. When the Thyroid Foundation of America recently asked treated patients how they felt, 59 percent still complained of muscle aches, lethargy and/or depression. Yet a study published in the *New England Journal of Medicine* found that when women with severe thyroid problems were treated with a T-4/T-3 combination, they felt a lot better.

Unfortunately, weight concerns weren't addressed in that particular study. So there's no way to know whether those women also lost weight. Still, Anita was on a T-4/T-3 regimen when she shed those 145 pounds. If your weight problems don't clear up with the first treatment you try, don't give up. Keep searching. You and your doctor may be able to fine-tune your options in some new way that will work great for you.

What about Diet and Exercise?

Exercise burns surprisingly few calories. But it will increase your fitness, raise your energy, reduce depression, and lower your stress levels. Strength training will also rebuild any muscle you may have lost during the thyroid imbalance. So the more you can get out and exercise, the better it will be for your health and your waistline. If you have trouble starting an exercise plan, go to Chapter 20, "Becoming an Exercise Winner."

As for diet, you'll obviously have to experiment. The best diet is the one you create for yourself. Still, you might want to start with an eating plan that eliminates sugars and starches and includes a bit more fat than the 30 percent the American Heart Association recommends. Why? Because many women with Lazy Thyroid Fat have other signs of the Deadly Quartet. If you're one of them, you may want to try what Stanford University endocrinologist Gerald Reaven calls his Syndrome X Diet. It's controversial, because it contains so much fat. But it's probably the most well-researched diet on the market if you have signs of the Deadly Quartet.

Basically, Reaven's theory is this: if you have high blood pressure, high triglycerides or other metabolic problems, you need to eat *more* dietary fat than normal to *lessen* your risks of heart disease, stroke, diabetes, and some cancers. Reaven recommends a diet that's a whopping 40 percent fat, most of it coming from soft margarine and "healthy" monosaturated fats like olive, walnut, and canola oils. Broda O. Barnes, M.D., a physician who studied hypothyroidism for more than thirty-five years and wrote a classic book titled *Hypothyroidism: The Unsuspected Illness* (still in print, but medically out of date), also hit on a diet for hypothyroidism very similar to the one Reaven describes. In short, many observant clinicians seem to have reached the same conclusion: a little extra fat in the diet leads to less around your middle—at least when Lazy Thyroid Fat is your problem.

What if you don't have any blood abnormalities? Then you may be able to lose weight safely on a diet that contains much less fat. Some winners with Lazy Thyroid Fat *do* report having lost weight on low-fat diets. Go to Chapter 19, "Designing Your Superconfidence Diet," for more information.

In the meantime, as you work to lose weight, watch your stress levels. Many doctors believe stress plays a bigger role in triggering and possibly prolonging thyroid problems than we've ever been told. In one German study published in *Psychiatry Research*, doctors measured TSH levels in East German refugees within six weeks of their arrival in Berlin shortly before or after the fall of the Berlin Wall. These people had experienced prolonged stress, with most of them suffering from anxiety, depression, and even post-traumatic stress disorders. A whopping 62 percent were in the hypothyroid range on the TSH test, although they showed no obvious clinical symptoms. Noting these abnormalities differed from those in depression, the researchers concluded their low thyroid functions were the result of "chronic stress." So even if you've corrected your hormone imbalance, be sure to go to Chapter 9, "Losing Daily Hassles Fat," to brainstorm for ways to calm down.

If you're struggling with depression, as women with Lazy Thyroid Fat frequently do, also go to Chapter 10, "Losing Depression Fat."

Finally, since Lazy Thyroid Fat and post-traumatic stress disorders often go hand in hand, see also Chapter 18, "Losing Post-Trauma Fat."

CHAPTER 12

Losing Anger Fat

If you are patient in one moment of anger, you will escape a hundred days of sorrow.

—Saying in a Chinese fortune cookie, quoted by Carol Tavris in Anger: The Misunderstood Emotion

When talk show host Rosie O'Donnell founded her Chub Club to encourage women of all weights to stay fit, she soon admitted feeling "imprisoned" by her own comments to start exercising more. "I was really stressed and angry that all these people were watching me and I had committed to doing this 5K," she recalls. When she got on the scale, she was shocked to see that since starting the Chub Club she'd gained 8 pounds and was now at her highest weight ever—216.

Why? Only O'Donnell can know for sure. But the anger she mentions couldn't have helped. In a group of 108 American women, those who reported more frequent angry feelings and outbursts and a sense of being unsupported by others were also more likely to have upper-body fat and other symptoms of the Deadly Quartet. Hostile and nonhostile men in a University of Utah study started out with similar cortisol levels when awakening in the morning. But as the day progressed, cynically hostile men had more than twice the increase in cortisol as more laid-back types.

This is a particularly unhealthy way to be fat. Anger Fat has been linked with high blood pressure, poor cholesterol profiles, and high insulin levels (all the major players in the Deadly Quartet). In one study of more than 5,000 people, angry women and men smoked more, drank more alcohol, and consumed 600 more calories on average a day than calmer types. Even worse, anger can *redistribute* your fat, storing more of it in your visceral danger zone, where it's been linked to all those diseases.

No one knows for sure how many overweight women struggle with Anger Fat, but the figures are high. In a series of Harvard Medical School studies led by Maurizio Fava, 31 percent of women with eating disorders (including anorexia and bingeing) and 48 percent of women struggling with depression experienced "anger attacks" (sudden spells of rapid heartbeats, hot flashes, and feelings of being out of control and wanting to attack others, followed by guilt or regret). Since anger has been strongly linked to heart disease, being angry *and* fat could put you at especially high risk. Duke University behavioral researcher Redford Williams estimates that 20 percent of us have hostility levels high enough to be hazardous to our hearts.

Is This Your Problem?

Mark a *T* for "true" or an *F* for "false" beside the following statements.

1. I often feel unsupported by those closest to me.
2. Anger is a powerful tool.
3. Most people would lie and cheat if they thought they could get away with it.
4. You can never trust anybody else to do the job right. You have to do it yourself.
5. In an argument, I'm usually the angrier one.
6. When someone treats you unfairly, it's hard to stop thinking about it.
7. It's good to get angry and tell people when they've been unfair, inept, or stupid. It's the only way to make them treat you with respect.
8. When somebody has an ignorant opinion or wastes my time, I tell them so. They need to be straightened out.
9. Little annoyances often get under my skin.
10. Just remembering my anger at someone can stir up my irritation again.

11. When I hear all the injustices in the news, I just want to lash out.
12. When I'm really angry, I slam doors or throw objects. On occasion, I've even shoved or hit people.

If you answered *true* to even two or three of these statements, you probably have Anger Fat. If you also eat, smoke, or drink alcohol when you're angry, you've probably already collected too much unhealthy fat in your visceral zone and need to get your anger under control.

The Most Fattening Ways to Be Angry

There are multiple ways to be angry, so many that scientists have only begun to sort them all out. Among the types of anger currently under investigation to see how they're connected with fat and/or disease are cynical, alienated, and powerless hostility; paranoia; suppressed anger; righteous indignation; cold, alienated anger; sullenness; grumpiness; irritability; neurotic anger; passive aggression; resentment; suspicion; aggressive behavior; and Machiavellianism. Then there's the hopeless, helpless anger called "vital exhaustion." People in this severe stage of anger are so overwhelmed with stress, they've almost burned out. They may flash angrily at the slightest frustration, yet also be "tired all the time."

If all these ways to be angry could kill us, we'd all be in trouble. Every time a rude motorist cut us off on the freeway or a broken vending machine kept our change, our waistlines would swell. Fortunately, only two ways to be angry have been connected so far to Anger Fat: cynical hostility (which includes pessimism and paranoia), and vital exhaustion.

Hostile anger, in particular, goes hand in hand with a host of unhealthy habits. Cynically hostile women and men smoke more, drink more, and eat unhealthier diets than less hostile people. In one study, highly hostile women consumed more animal fat, less fiber, and more cholesterol than mellower women did. Hostile men also ate more sugar and took in lower levels of calcium than their calmer counterparts.

Does hostility cause people to crave fat? Does anger somehow promote smoking—or, conversely, does smoking give you a short fuse? Though scientists haven't answered these questions, you—as the curious scientist of your own body—can certainly answer them for yourself. What's your experience? Do you crave fat or a cigarette when you're angry? Do certain ways of expressing your anger stimulate your appetite more than other ways do? Do you eat only before—or only after—you've blown your top? Try keeping an anger diary for a while to see what insights you gain.

Breaking the Anger Trap

Unfortunately, our whole culture has an "anger problem." We don't "do anger" well. Whether it's Peter Finch in that old movie *Network* screaming out the window, "I'm mad as hell and I'm not going to take it anymore," two trucks racing each other down the freeway in road rage, or troubled teens shooting up their high school in Colorado, we have poor role models for coping with our frustrations. The first step toward losing Anger Fat, therefore, involves learning to handle anger better than you have before. Here's a cafeteria of strategies you can try to get your anger and waistline back under control:

1. USE ANGER TO TAKE CHARGE

We're often told to control our anger. But it's more important to express anger in ways that make us *feel* in control. When it comes to developing unhealthy fat, two ways of handling anger—"anger out" and "anger in"—have garnered special attention. When you're in an *anger-out* mode, you make sarcastic remarks, slam doors, hurl saucepans or insults, and strike out at whatever or whomever is handy. In an *anger-in* state, you sulk, pout, harbor a secret grudge, or silently "boil inside" without showing it.

Is it more fattening to suppress anger—or to just explode and get it all off your chest? Most of us would vote against suppression. We're told not to hold in our feelings. So here's a big surprise. They're *both* fattening. In one large study of women, *anger-out* was the culprit. Frequently hostile women who let everyone "have it" also had higher levels of visceral fat. Yet *anger-in* can also be fattening, especially when it leads to vital exhaustion.

Why would expressing anger be just as fattening as holding it in? As you'll recall from Frankenhaeuser's work, the key to feeling less stress is feeling more in control. Tossing pans and storming around the house may *look* liberated to an intimidated bystander (often a child), but the raging woman may secretly feel quite out of control. In the Women's Anger Study being conducted at the University of Tennessee, many women's anger began as a confusing mixture of feelings, such as hurt, frustration, and disappointment. Once women finally realized they were angry, those who submissively kept quiet (anger in) and those who "let it all hang out" in a furious outburst (anger out) felt *equally powerless*. The women who blew their stacks saw their anger as a distressful loss of control.

Fortunately, there's a third choice that's best for your waist and your health: using your anger calmly but effectively to gain others' respect. In the Women's Anger Study, women reported a sense of power and control only when they used anger to restore justice, respect, and equality in their relationships.

So the next time you feel ravenous, take a ten-minute break. You may be in that muddled pre-anger phase, right before you fully realize why you're upset. Review what happened in the last ten or twelve hours. Did your mate hurt your feelings? Did your mother chide you about being fat? Were you playing martyr again? Once you figure out why you're upset, brainstorm for ways you'd like to see the problem resolved. You may need to tell your mother firmly but calmly that you appreciate her concern, but your weight is your problem. It's liberating to let people know you're angry, so long as you do it in a powerful, *solution-focused* way that increases your sense of control. Raging often only backfires and makes you feel more helpless.

2. LEARN HOW TO SAY NO

Anger Fat frequently springs from the fact you're overwhelmed by chores that matter very little to you. Straining to meet everyone else's needs, you forget to take care of your own. So how do you say no to others' requests without feeling that tug of guilt or that lump in your throat?

Books and classes on assertiveness training offer countless ideas on the best ways to say no. But when we examine how the winners manage to say no to requests, one theme keeps emerging. Lonnie, a happy 170-pound girls' basketball coach, put it well: "Realize you're worthwhile. You were put here for a purpose, and what *you* do matters." The ability to say no—and to control your weight—springs from the robust kind of self-confidence that comes from knowing you're lovable and "nice" just as you are, and you don't have to buy love by dutifully caving in to everybody else's requests.

How does exercising your best talents help you say no? "I used to be a real wimp, the classic patsy," Lonnie says. "I'd say yes to any time-consuming project or chore anyone asked me to do, then I'd get angry because I felt so put upon. One day I realized I needed to become more fully involved in what mattered most to me. While I'm coaching, I'm not just teaching basketball. I encourage these girls to assert themselves and go after their dreams. One girl I coached was on the verge of becoming anorexic. I told her the truth: she lacked energy on the court because she wasn't eating enough. She gained 20 pounds, became our star forward, and just won a college basketball scholarship. Now because I'm doing what *I* feel is important, I have no trouble turning down others' insistent requests. I find when I'm saying yes to my own truths, it's very easy to say no to someone else's unfair demands."

In her own "winner's way," Lonnie has achieved what assertiveness coach Manuel J. Smith (author of *When I Say No, I Feel Guilty*) calls the prime right that keeps anyone from manipulating you: "the right to be the final judge of yourself."

3. ANGER-PROOF YOUR RELATIONSHIP

Nothing can perpetuate Anger Fat more than a hostile relationship. Being constantly furious at your mate keeps Anger Fat building day after day. In one survey of 9,000 women, those who'd been unhappily married for thirteen years had gained an average of 42½ pounds. If you find yourself constantly complaining because that "damned man" refuses to tell you how he's feeling, weasels out of the housework, blames you for everything, denies your feelings, constantly needles you, makes weekend plans without consulting you, flirts with other women at parties, _____ (you fill in the blank), realize this: he may never reform. But you may get fat.

Does this mean if you want to get thin that you can never air a grievance or that you always have to "fight nice"? Fortunately, no. Now that therapists have begun studying strong, healthy relationships (not just troubled couples who wind up in therapy), they're finding that even happy couples—the relationship "winners"—sometimes have loud screaming matches. Even in good marriages that have lasted for years, University of Washington psychologist John Gottman reports, 80 percent of the time men pull the old "silent treatment" routine, refusing to discuss problems. You don't need a picture-perfect marriage to be happy—or thin.

But you do need to keep cynical hostility under control. Here's how couples in happy, resilient relationships often handle their differences. Maybe some of these tips will help you rethink anger in your relationship.

- Agree to disagree. We've been taught every marital problem has a solution. Wrong. Gottman videotaped happily married people fighting over one major issue of their own choice; four years later, he videotaped them again. An amazing 69 percent of these happy couples were still fighting about the *same problem* in the same way! Gottman says, "When you marry, you automatically inherit your set of unresolvable relationship problems. If you married somebody else, you'd have a different set. It just comes with the territory."
- Solve problems as a team. If you keep spinning your wheels over a power struggle, try sitting down calmly and working out the problem together. Instead of seeing the issue as *his* problem that *he* needs to fix, see it as a problem *both* of you share and need to address. If you've been fighting about money for years, maybe you can find some solutions together.
- Express needs directly. *Be specific.* If you want sympathy or an hour alone, say so. Don't get angry when people can't read your mind. Also, aim for concrete solutions. If he frequently leaves you waiting in a restaurant bar for two hours, would his being *one hour* late be okay? Or would you like for him to phone if he's even fifteen minutes delayed? Merely airing grievances gets you nowhere.
- Choose your battles. You may be able to tolerate his dirty socks on the floor but go crazy when he insults your mother. Continual bickering over *every* issue only keeps your marriage in turmoil. It may also keep you fat.

- When hashing it out, don't resort to angry sulking, crying, threatening to leave, throwing saucepans, or sarcastic name-calling. Stick to the point. If the issue is his gambling and he retorts, "Well, you eat too much" or worse, "You're a fat pig," ignore his counter-attack and reply calmly, "My weight is my problem, and I'm working on that. Right now we're talking about your gambling."
- Don't gripe about his faults to others. We're often told that airing our anger and "getting anger off our chests" will cool it down. That old "ventilation theory" of anger (which dates to the 1950s) has long been disproved. In reality, complaining about your relationship to your sister, best friend, or mother usually only *rehearses* anger and makes it flame hotter.
- Use your sense of humor. One winner married thirty-eight years knows this trick well. "Mark and I turn arguments into laughs all the time," she told me. How? "Look at the big picture and ask, 'What's to be gained here by holding on to my viewpoint?' You'll realize life is too short. It just isn't worth it."
- Finally, realize that if you can "fall out of love," you can also "fall out of hate." Happy couples do it all the time. You may also want to pick up a few good books on improving marital communication, such as *The Dance of Anger* by Harriet Lerner or *You Just Don't Understand* by Deborah Tannen.

4. LEARN TO FORGIVE

If you're chronically angry and have the spare tire to prove it, you may have genuine reason. Sometimes life *is* "unjust." But it's even more unfair to punish *yourself* for others' crimes by eating to stifle your rage.

When you forgive, you're not letting the other guy off the hook. You're not condoning injustice. You're merely saying, "I will not allow myself to hurt by this act any longer." Forgiveness doesn't mean going back for more brutal treatment. You don't even have to mend your relationship with the person who hurt you. You simply have to *stop hurting*.

If just my saying this makes you enraged, you've probably been hurt very deeply and Chapter 18, "Losing Post-Trauma Fat," may be for you. You may inwardly scream, "What do you think I've been trying to do all these years? I'd love nothing more than to stop hurting, but I can't." Remember this: *forgiveness means letting go of pain.* Or if you prefer, *letting go of your desire for revenge.* That's it. That's all it is. What's more, letting go of pain or a desire for revenge is a technique you can learn. Letting go of pain is a skill.

One of the best books on forgiveness I've read is *Exploring Forgiveness,* edited by Robert Enright of the University of Wisconsin–Madison and Joanna North, a philosophy teacher at the University of London. (Archbishop Desmond Tutu wrote the introduction.) Enright believes so much in the power of forgiveness, he's founded the International Forgiveness Institute to stimulate research in this area. One of the salient points in this book is that there's a clear difference between true and "false" forgiveness. If we "forgive" someone but then continually remind them how much they hurt us and expect them to be eternally indebted to us, Enright and his colleagues say, "we are exercising a superiority that is incompatible with forgiveness." Superficial forgiveness, in which we "forgive" but also secretly hold onto the rage, is also false. True forgiveness, the kind that heals the pain, is often a long journey. You should never be rushed into it. You must be ready.

There are many barriers to forgiveness, not the least of which are anger, fear, mistrust, and having had parents who never showed us how to do it. But as Philadelphia psychiatrist Richard Fitzgibbons notes, forgiveness has "remarkable healing powers," including better anger control, a greater capacity to love and trust, more confidence, better sleep patterns, and even fewer physical illnesses. It can also help you lose fat. When you release an old pain and give up your desire for revenge, people around you (particularly your children and spouse) may even become less anxious and stressed. Forgiveness, which we're often taught to view as a weakness, is actually a great strength in disguise.

CHAPTER 13

Losing Two Kinds of Binge-Eating Fat

While Japanese people have said "eat till 80% full," Polynesian cultures have said, "eat until tired." . . . We must retrain ourselves to learn another standard of eating that differs from what our culture has taught us.

*—Julie Gast and Steven R. Hawks,
University of Utah*

To everyone who knows her, forty-one-year-old Claire is an enviably stylish, talented, successful advertising executive, the kind of picture-perfect woman who has it all. But for years in her private life, Claire had a dark secret:

It usually started when I was home alone and thinking about some forbidden food I was dying to eat but had denied myself for weeks—like buttered popcorn, homemade chocolate fudge, or ice cream. I'd start obsessing about it, and before long that's all I could think about. Finally, I'd get so tired of my mind spinning around, I'd give in and tell myself, "Oh, go ahead. You can have it. You've been good. If you eat it now, you'll relax." So I'd go into the kitchen and make a batch of chocolate fudge or a huge bowl of popcorn swimming in butter. Then I'd sit down alone and start eating.

At first, I'd nibble slowly, just savoring every bite. If it was popcorn, I'd eat one buttery, salty kernel at a time. Mmmm. Delicious. But then before I knew it, I'd begin eating faster and faster, almost as if I was in a trance, totally out of control. I'd gorge myself until my stomach ached. Afterward, I'd feel guilty, bloated, and fat. I kept telling myself, "This is insane. I'm a smart woman with a college degree, a man who loves me, and a terrific career. So why do I do such stupid things to myself?"

If you can identify with Claire's secret life, you're not alone. Millions of women, including about 25 to 30 percent who attend weight-loss clinics, have Binge-Eating Syndrome. "A generation ago, the term *binge* meant one thing to most people: drinking to excess. Today the word more often means eating to excess," says Christopher G. Fairburn, a noted binge-eating authority at the University of Oxford.

Everybody has dietary lapses. From time to time, we all over-indulge. But Binge-Eating Syndrome differs from a garden-variety splurge in two ways: first, you eat a lot more in a set period of time (say, one or two hours) than most people would eat during that same period under the same circumstances. Bingers have been known eat as many as 12,000 calories at a sitting, though 2,000 is more typical. Second, you feel out of control and unable to stop.

This distressful sense of being *out of control* is the key to a true binge. Other signs you're struggling with Binge-Eating Syndrome include feeling tense, depressed, and guilty after you've eaten; wolfing down food so fast you barely have time to chew (in one Columbia University study, bingers ate more than twice as many calories per minute as nonbingers); hiding the problem from friends and family (it's your dirty little secret); and possibly going into a "trance" or "numbing out" as you eat. (In this latter case, you may also have Post-Trauma Fat and may want to read Chapter 18 in conjunction with this one.)

Since eating too much at times is the hallmark of this syndrome, isn't being overweight also a symptom? Not necessarily. Many thin women also binge, but then "purge" to undo the damage of all that food by dieting severely, fasting for days, vomiting, or compulsively exercising. Some female runners starve themselves, eating as little as 1,000 calories a day before a race, then binge afterwards on a huge meal of 6,000 calories or more. (Purging *before* you binge is called *debting*.) If you use any of these forms of purging, you have what's called Bulimia Nervosa (BN). People may even remark that you have no weight problem (but you secretly know that you do). If you don't purge, you have a more recently defined condition called Binge-Eating Disorder (BED). In this second case, since you do nothing to offset your eating, you're probably overweight and carrying around too much visceral fat.

The myth that all fat people overeat may have sprung from studies of women with Binge-Eating Fat. Bingers *do* overeat—at least some of the time. If you have Bulimia Nervosa, however, you may also *undereat* at other times. Often it's both the overeating *and* the undereating that eventually make you fat. They're connected, tied together as inextricably as the rise and fall of an ocean wave. Wholeness requires that we be in balance and in touch with the deep, subtle rhythms of our mind/body/spirits. Bingers are so jangled by stress, they're out of balance. That's why their eating patterns are so erratic . . . and erratic eating patterns, in turn, feed back into stress.

Is This Your Problem?

1. Do you eat lots of food rapidly in a short amount of time—then feel really guilty and distressed afterward?
2. Do you try to "undo" the damage of all that food you've eaten by exercising or dieting obsessively or even vomiting?
3. Do you often feel bloated, fat, stuffed, and miserable after overeating?
4. When you start eating some foods, do you become afraid you can't stop?

If you answered yes to any of these questions, you may have Binge-Eating Syndrome. If you also answered yes to question 2, you have what's called Bulimia Nervosa, a special subtype of this disorder.

Finding Your Way to Take Charge

Although one driving force behind bingeing is low confidence around food, that's no problem. Happily, rhythmic superconfidence is a craft you can learn. How? By developing skills. If you're overweight, you need to acknowledge that you don't have just one problem. You have two: the bingeing *and* the weight. By its very definition, Binge-Eating Fat is a nesting syndrome. First you have to stop bingeing. That's your top priority. Then—and only then—can you begin to slim down. So let's set aside how to get thin for a minute and examine the skills that will help you get back in charge.

1. FIND YOUR TRUE TRIGGERS

You'll often hear that the best way to beat a binge is to keep all "trigger foods" out of the house. Out of sight, out of mind. It makes perfect sense. Problem is, if you binge on many different foods or shop for groceries so you *can* binge, avoiding just one or two foods like ice cream or doughnuts won't help. You need to probe deeper.

Many bingers report it's not really food that triggers their binges, anyway. It's negative feelings. In an eating disorders clinic in Sydney, Australia, a whopping 91 percent of binge eaters named "tension" as a binge trigger. Other common triggers include loneliness, anger, boredom, sadness, "visiting my parents," arriving home tired from work, feeling inadequate or helpless after an ego blow, having PMS, and drinking alcohol.

When searching for your own truths, think of a trigger in terms of a *pattern*. "A trigger is not just an on/off switch," note internationally known eating-disorder specialists Johan Vanderlinden and Walter Vandereycken of Belgium. They add that "a careful analysis often reveals a kind of 'automatic' scenario." First, you may feel angry, depressed, or lonely. Then you think about food. Then you may have to go grocery shopping. Then you return home and arrange to be alone so no one can watch you, and so on. Carefully examine your binge patterns (record your observations in a journal). You'll soon see that what you thought was a totally "unpredictable" loss of control is, in fact, a highly predictable chain of events. Decide which links in the chain you can change.

Claire (the woman at the start of this chapter) realized her binges usually began when she was home alone and started obsessing about food. Her chain then continued when she entered the kitchen and whipped up a batch of fudge or popcorn. She chose to break the chain at the get-go by interrupting her obsessive thoughts. Instead of allowing her mind to start "spinning around" without direction as she obsessed about food, she wrote down a list of things she could do when she was at risk of losing control:

- Call a friend, your sister, or brother.
- Take a bubble bath and meditate to relax.
- Listen to music or a self-hypnosis tape on your Walkman.
- Stroll down to the library and check out a book.
- Rapidly write down all your feelings and thoughts in your journal.
- Go out for a brisk walk.
- If it's raining, jump rope or lift weights.
- Start painting, drawing, writing, or knitting.
- Take thirty deep, deep breaths.

Armed with this detailed self-generated list, which she kept posted on a bulletin board in her study and also on the refrigerator door, she was gradually able to see which strategies worked best for her. The ones that worked she kept doing. The ones that didn't work she discarded. She beat her binge eating eight years ago. During the subsequent year she lost 22 pounds. See "Seven Quick Binge Busters" on page 150 for more great binge busters.

Are You a Food Addict?

One recovering alcoholic became such a compulsive overeater she gained 100 pounds in less than a year. Tormented, she began weeping while telling a friend, "You have no idea what torture it is to be a food junkie. When you're hooked on alcohol, you can go cold turkey. But when you're addicted to food, you can never kick the habit, because you *have* to eat."

This unhappy woman is certainly compulsive and deserves help. But is she truly "addicted" with no hope for relief? Thankfully, the latest science says no. In our society, we often use the word *addict* so loosely (as in sex addict, love addict, TV junkie) that it's easy to get confused. To be a true addiction, a substance must create a *biological* dependency, the way alcohol does. Oxford University's Christopher G. Fairburn, arguably the world's leading binge-eating expert, calls the notion of overeating as an addiction a "far-fetched" myth "not supported by facts." No evidence has ever shown bingeing results from a biological abnormality, he observes. What's more, the most successful ways to cure bingeing often differ 180 degrees from the twelve-step approach that works so well in programs like Alcoholics Anonymous. In AA, recovering alcoholics are taught, "The disease never gets better. It gets worse unless you *immediately* abstain." With Binge-Eating Syndrome, full recoveries are quite common, and slow, steady, gradual changes work just as well as abrupt stopping. Rather than viewing any food as "toxic" (a kind of all-or-nothing thinking, which has no basis in fact), you need to learn that no food is poison.

This is why most "forbidden food" diets are especially bad for binge eaters. When you're a binger and try to avoid a whole class of foods (like fats or sugar, and other carbs), you could even flip over and become anorexic, an outcome you might find "attractive in principle but a nightmare in reality," Fairburn notes. When struggling with Binge-Eating Fat, you've already been beaten up quite enough by your own guilt and remorse (and possibly a childhood history of sexual abuse). In place of a blitzkrieg "succeed or die" diet, you need and deserve a gentler, much more loving approach laced with self-understanding and self-forgiveness.

2. KICK THE DIET HABIT

You'll often hear "diets don't work." This statement comes largely from the binge-eating literature. Why? Because for you diets *don't* work. In fact, they may only make your problem worse. In one British study, young women currently on diets were *eight times* more likely to develop binge-eating problems during the subsequent year. So in some women strict dieting may not only perpetuate this problem, it may also cause it.

Unfortunately, telling a binge eater to stop dieting is like telling a bungee jumper to cut the cord. Diets for you may be a survival tool to deal with stress. The fact that they haven't *worked* for you (if they did, why aren't you stress-free?) often goes overlooked in your struggle to get back in charge.

Counterintuitive as it sounds, to stop bingeing, you must stop dieting. You must normalize your eating behavior. How? First, you need to start with a plan that for you may be very abnormal: you need to eat three planned meals plus two or three planned snacks every day. "Oh, my God," you may think. "With all that food, I'd blow up like a balloon." I told you it would sound counterintuitive. But trust me on this. This will keep you from getting hungry and possibly rev up your metabolism, which by now may really be out of whack.

Dr. Fairburn, who has had a *90 percent success rate* with this program and wrote a highly recommended self-help book titled *Overcoming Binge Eating*, suggests this typical pattern:

8 A.M.: Breakfast
10:30 A.M.: Midmorning snack
12:30 P.M.: Lunch
3:30 P.M.: Midafternoon snack
7:00 P.M.: Dinner or supper
9:00 P.M.: Evening snack

You may not be hungry at all these times. But eat anyway. We're often told to "listen to our bodies" and follow our natural appetites. This sounds like sensible advice. But when you're a binge eater, your body's signals are often so jangled they're no longer reliable guides. To eliminate chaotic eating, you need to go *no more* than three or four hours between feedings.

How could you possibly eat all the food this guy recommends? Remember, you don't have to eat giant amounts at any one sitting. In fact, that's the idea. Your snack might be just a cup of juice or an apple. One winner who had a bagel as part of her breakfast saved half of it for her midmorning snack. Still, at this point, Fairburn notes, it's not *what* you eat but *when* that's most crucial. Even if you binge, try not to cut down the size of your next snack or meal. But won't you gain weight by eating so often? Probably not. In fact, oddly enough, you may lose. For one thing, you'll rev up your metabolism when you eat more regularly. For another, you'll be less tempted to binge, so you'll never eat a huge amount rapidly at any one time.

Other tips that can help:

- Formalize your eating. Always sit down at the table (don't eat on the sofa or in the bedroom). Never eat standing up.

- Focus on eating (don't read a book or watch TV). Stay "mindful" (see "Observe Your Thoughts" on page 94). Eat slowly and deliberately, tasting each bite.
- When eating in a restaurant or with friends, avoid alcohol (which can lead to a binge) and keep an eye on the different courses. You may even want to skip a course or two, so you can keep better track of what you've eaten without going overboard. Don't let others pressure you to eat more than you planned. This is your show.

Over time, your binges will lessen, your metabolism will stabilize, and you may very well lose weight naturally as a side effect of restoring your normal biological rhythms.

If the above program sounds too rigid for you, remember it was designed for women with *serious* binge problems, the ones who show up in clinics. If you have less serious problems, you may be able to modify this plan in a way that would work better for you. But however serious or minor your problem, the *principles* for solving it are the same. Restoring your natural rhythms and eliminating chaotic eating (along with ferreting out triggers and reducing stress) can contribute greatly to your solutions.

Did winners who beat Binge-Eating Fat do it the way Fairburn describes? They often did, but it frequently took them years to hit on this solution. Connie, a TV producer who finally overcame a serious twenty-year binge habit on her own, says, "It dawned on me one day that my eating was so erratic it just had to be bad for my psychological, physical, and spiritual health. I was also getting fatter every year. I'd alternate between paying no attention at all to food for days, then pigging out like a madwoman. At first I hated thinking about food three times a day (and even five times when I considered snacks). It seemed like a colossal waste of my precious time. With my high-pressure job, I'm constantly on the run and tend to be immensely impatient. But once I realized how much calmer I felt, I knew the effort was worthwhile." Margot, another recovered binger, says: "Learning to eat more regularly was like learning to exercise. For years, I never exercised. I felt miserable and depressed but didn't know why. Once I started swimming and mountain hiking regularly, my spirits rose. Now when I skip my exercise, I really miss it. The same's true with my eating. Now I have to eat regularly, because when I do, I feel so energetic and happy. Regular habits really keep my stress levels down."

Seven Quick Binge Busters

These tactics have all worked for weight-control winners. Try them. Invent your own variations. Experiment until you find what works best for you.

1. When you feel like bingeing, do an "emotion check." Ask, "How am I feeling right now—and *why*?" Why are you angry, scared, anxious, or threatened? Rapidly "free-write" your thoughts and feelings in a large, spiral notebook. You may be amazed what insights emerge.
2. Create a "safe place" fantasy: a beautiful wildflower meadow, a peaceful country lane, a wooded glen with a pool and gentle waterfall. "Go there" in your mind when you feel a binge coming on.
3. Call a friend who knows about your problem and just have her listen. Picture a loved one's face. If you're devoutly religious, picture Jesus, Moses, the Blessed Mother, the Dalai Lama, or the Buddha.
4. Take ten, twenty, or a hundred deep, cleansing breaths. Tune in to your breathing and focus on the rhythms of your breath. In-out, in-out, like ocean waves. Feel the soothing of your own breathing, almost as if you're being rocked gently in a great big rocking chair.
5. Brush your teeth so your mouth feels clean. Dump food in the garbage disposal or soak it with water.
6. Get a dog. One winner says, "When I feel like bingeing, walking the dog gives me a chance to get out of the house and exercise without feeling alone."
7. Swim, dance to your favorite music, go for a bike ride. In one survey, 80 percent of Binge-Eating Syndrome winners said moderate exercise "provided a break from emotional pressures." One winner said, "I jog, but I expect any kind of exercise will do if it works up a good, honest sweat."

---

3. FACE DOWN FOOD FEARS

Fears about food run rampant in our culture. We're continually told fat is "bad," carbohydrates are "bad," white bread is "bad," red meat is "bad," egg yolks are "bad" (the whites are okay), caffeine is "really bad," and sugar is more than bad: it's downright "toxic." Fettucine Alfredo, that creamy, delectable pleasure, has been dubbed the "heart attack on a plate." Even dairy products have been branded as deadly. Many aggressively marketed fad diets are really just "fear-your-food" diets. Apparently, their designers figure if you're scared out of your wits, you won't eat. But as a binger, *you* know that fear only makes you eat more.

To stop bingeing for life, you need to rid yourself of false food fears and ignore fear mongers for profit. *Unless it's rotten, no food is inherently bad.* Even chocolate contains antioxidants (disease-fighting plant chemicals) that may combat cancer. What about allergies? Okay, sure, a few of us have allergies or genetic problems digesting some foods (those with celiac sprue disease need to avoid wheat, for example). But such conditions are rare. The vast majority of women are not allergic to our dinner plates or anything on them. If you've been convinced you're "addicted" to certain foods as if they were some kind of drug, see "Are You a Food Addict?" on page 146.

Brenda, who once never allowed herself doughnuts except on a binge, overcame her food fears by going once a week to a bakery and buying just one doughnut, then taking it home and eating at the kitchen table. She really focused on enjoying the taste. Afterward, she wrote all her feelings in a notebook (her journal): she recorded how eating the doughnut made her feel, what thoughts she had as she ate it, how she felt afterward, and so on. To ensure this "fearful" doughnut wouldn't trigger a major binge, she always planned something to do right after she ate it (such as visiting her best friend, practicing the piano for an hour, or picking up her son from soccer practice). Slowly, she was able to gain control and eat one doughnut without guilt or self-blame.

Arlene had several foods on her "forbidden" list, but her number one villain was chocolate ice cream. Once she started eating it, she felt helplessly unable to stop until she consumed the whole quart or half-gallon.

"I realized I almost had an ice cream phobia," she recalls. "So I decided to take fear apart and face it head-on. First, I made a list detailing all the things surrounding ice cream that made me anxious: from just thinking about eating it to going on a full-fledged binge. Then I practiced meditating quietly, as I pictured ice cream in my mind. I'd visualize myself opening the carton, dipping a spoon in the ice cream, etc., just like a little movie. As I ran this little movie in my mind, I'd notice my thoughts. When I'd become anxious and almost start to hyperventilate, I'd calm myself down with deep breathing. Then I'd continue to visualize the ice cream. I did this every day for about two weeks."

Her next step was to go to the supermarket (with a friend for support) and walk down the ice cream aisle until she could do it without getting anxious. She recalls, "I'd practice breath focus." (This is a technique described in Chapter 9, "Losing Daily Hassles Fat.") Since she's devoutly religious, she also prayed to God to help her succeed. Once she was able to walk past the ice cream case calmly, she stopped one day in front of it but didn't buy anything. Each time she was able to beat her fears and achieve one small victory, her confidence rose. Gradually, step by step, she was able to quell her anxieties and reduce her stress to the point where she was able to buy one quart of chocolate Häagen-Dazs, eat half a cup, then leave the rest in the freezer. Now whenever she buys ice cream, it often sits in her fridge for days before she even thinks about it.

Arlene laughs. "Some people might think that sounds like an awful lot of work just to 'beat' a bowl of ice cream. But what really matters is that I had a major problem, I confronted it head-on, and I solved it my way." You might want to try your variation of Arlene's solution. Or you might devise an entirely different strategy. The important point is to *try something*. Once you know what works, do more of it. If an idea doesn't pan out, try something else.

4. FOCUS ON WALKING THE TIGHTROPE

When you have Binge-Eating Fat, it's easy to fret about all the ways you can mess up. "I'm so uptight that when I get home from work tonight, I'd better not look at that cherry pie or even *think* about the ice cream in the refrigerator. Otherwise, I'm bound to pig out." Focusing on all the ways you can *avoid failure* rather than on the one way you can *succeed* sets you up for a fall. In *Leaders: The Strategies for Taking Charge* (a book about winners in business), professors Warren Bennis and Burt Nanus tell the story of the famous aerialist Karl

Wallenda, who fell to his death in 1978 after walking a 75-foot high wire in Puerto Rico. His wife (also an aerialist) recalled: "All Karl thought about for three straight months prior to [that walk] was *falling*. It was the first time he'd ever thought about that, and it seemed to me that he put all his energies into *not falling* rather than walking the tightrope." Bennis and Nanus write: "From what we learned from our interviews with successful leaders, it became increasingly clear that when Wallenda poured his energies into *not falling* rather than walking the tightrope, he was virtually destined to fall."

From what I learned from interviewing weight-control winners, I totally agree. When you focus on problems, you see only problems. When you focus on solutions, you see only solutions. To become superconfident when tackling your binge eating, map out your solution plan, then focus singlemindedly on the best way you know to do the job *right* (Example: "When I get home from work, I'll immediately change into my sweatpants and go out for a run. Afterward, I'll take a shower, then call Sarah to see if she wants to go to the mall. If she's busy, I'll go shopping alone. When I get tired, I'll come home and go straight to bed.")

5. ASK THE MIRACLE QUESTION

You may believe you "always" binge. But, in fact, nothing *always* happens. There are always exceptions. To find those exceptions, some therapists are having great success with what's called "the miracle question." Here's how it works: imagine that when you go to bed tonight while you're sleeping, a "miracle" happens and your binge eating problem is solved. Presto! Just like that. Since you were sleeping, you weren't aware the miracle happened. When you wake up tomorrow morning, what's the first small thing you'll notice that will tell you the miracle has happened and your binge-eating problem is solved? Your answers will help you discover surprising new strengths.

Barbara McFarland, a therapist at the Eating Disorders Recovery Center in Cincinnati, frequently asks this question to help binge eaters zero in on their goals. In answer to the question above, one woman who eventually became a winner said:

> *I would not be thinking of what I was going to have for breakfast. I would be thinking, instead, about things I was going to get done. . . . I'd eat the*

right kinds of foods and want to. I'd have a bagel and juice for breakfast and a salad with my fat-free dressing on it for lunch. I'd be going to exercise and excited about it. I'd be happier. I'd dress up like I used to. The way I used to be. My husband would know the miracle had happened because he'd see me out of the house, going to the gym every morning, calling up friends and asking them to do things.

Just focusing on her solutions was enough to get her headed in the right direction. Soon she was going to the gym every morning.

When asked when she most recently had a "miracle day" or anything close to it, another woman who eventually beat her binge eating told McFarland about a day she and her husband were on vacation. What was different about that day? What made it "better" than her binge days? "We got up early and took a walk down the beach. I was so relaxed and happy. We first had breakfast, and I had a really healthy one. Some fat-free yogurt with this fabulous fresh fruit, a bagel with fat-free cream cheese, and coffee." Asked if having a healthy breakfast was different for her, she replied, "Oh, gosh, yes. I usually don't eat breakfast at all." The lesson this winner took from her miracle day was that eating a healthy breakfast made the rest of her day better—and kept her from bingeing.

What are the "exceptions" in your life? When does your bingeing *not* happen? By carefully describing those times to a friend or jotting them in a journal, you'll find more solutions than you ever imagined.

Do You Have a Body Image Problem?

Some women who binge secretly long to be enviably *superthin* (not fit and healthy). The more you believe "what is fat is bad, what is thin is beautiful, and what is beautiful is good or likely to increase your odds of professional success," the more you may also be vulnerable to bingeing and purging, possibly by becoming what leading eating-disorders authority Judith Rodin calls a "workout-aholic." If you're healthy but still want to be thinner just for looks *no matter what*, you may want to read (or reread) a few feminist books like Naomi Wolf's *The Beauty Myth* or Susie Orbach's *Fat Is a Feminist*

Issue. Fat, of course, isn't *always* a feminist issue. If you have Lazy Thyroid, PCOS, or Medication-Caused Fat, to cite just three examples, it's clearly a medical problem. But for some binge eaters, becoming more informed about cultural pressures on women can be an alternative to feeling distressed.

6. BECOME YOUR OWN GOOD MOM

Some binge eating may have its roots in a troubled childhood. Binge eaters frequently report the death of a parent, family alcoholism, or childhood sexual abuse. As a child, when you felt scared, lonely, or sad, you may have learned to soothe yourself in the best way you knew how (with food), and somehow the pattern stuck. Jane, who finally gained the skills to stop bingeing after struggling for ten years, recalls many dinnertimes when her alcoholic mother was passed out on the sofa. Having to fend for herself (she was only three or four at the time), Jane frequently made her own "dinners" out of cookies, ice cream, and crackers. When she grew up and became angry or scared, she binged on, guess what? Cookies, ice cream, and crackers.

As a child, Jane was displaying her resilience and strength (how many three-year-olds can make their own dinner?). But as a grown woman, she longed to find healthier ways to deal with distress. She believes her recovery began the day she vowed to start taking care of the scared little girl inside her by "rewiring her brain." She began eliminating old mental ruts ("you're stupid, selfish, ugly, etc.") by replacing them with new thought patterns like, "You're doing well. That was a great job you did. You're really smart, you know that?" She literally wrote down a list of things she always wished her mother would have told her and began *saying* them. Slowly, the low-level depression she'd struggled with for years began lifting, and her urges to binge disappeared.

The strategy Jane hit on through trial and learning was much like a tool psychologists call "cognitive restructuring" or eliminating "negative self-talk." Here are some ways to free yourself from old no-confidence ruts and gain the superconfidence you need to take charge.

Replace conditional with unconditional love. Old no-confidence rut: I'll love you *if* you're a success, *if* you make the grade, *if* you don't talk back, *if* you brush your hair, *if* you're thin, *if* you're "good."

Superconfident new pattern: I'll always love you *whether or not* you're a success, *whether or not* you make the grade, *whether or not* you clean up the house, *whether or not* you've had time to brush your hair, *whether or not* you're thin.

Look at the big picture. Old no-confidence rut: I binged on Friday night. I blew it all. That one night just reflects my whole shitty life. All my good intentions are shot.

Superconfident new pattern: I binged Friday night, but I didn't binge at all on Saturday or Sunday. What can I learn about my success on Saturday and Sunday that I can use the next time I feel a binge coming on?

See mistakes as "solutions in progress." Old no-confidence rut: I binged on Friday night. This is just the same old thing over and over again. My life will never change.

Superconfident new pattern: Life is a process of constant change, and I'm changing right now. I didn't binge on Saturday or Sunday. That was something new, a success I need to hold onto. I wonder what else I can learn from that slipup on Friday.

Replace all-or-nothing thinking with problem solving. Old no-confidence rut: I felt lousy on Friday night because my whole life is lousy. If I keep bingeing like this, nobody will ever love me.

Superconfident new pattern: I felt lousy on Friday night because it had been a long week, and I was tired. The next time I'm tired, I think I'll take a hot bubble bath, give myself a neck massage, go to bed early, and read a juicy mystery until I drift off to sleep.

Take full responsibility (for victories as well as slipups). Old no-confidence rut: No wonder I binged. I have a lousy job, and my boss is a jerk. He's just like my dad, always so high and mighty, like he knows it all. I hate all men.

Superconfident new pattern: Bingeing was a free choice that I made, and I know that. I also made the choice on Saturday and Sunday *not* to binge. It felt good being in charge.

7. Dismiss Slipups as Flukes

The unconfident among us tend to overdramatize—and personalize—gaffes. When we overeat, we say, "I can't believe I ate all that. How can I be so stupid? I never do anything right." The superconfident winner simply says, "Oops." Winners may have "screwups," "glitches," or "foul-ups." But they never actually *fail*. Operating from what therapists Lindsey Hall and Leigh Cohn call "a framework of success rather than failure," they simply use setback binges as a chance to better understand their compulsions. "In every person's case," Hall and Cohn found when they studied winners, "recovery meant taking action, enduring emotional pressures, and having some binges during the early stages of healing." One winner, who once had a full-blown case of bingeing with vomiting, said she used her setbacks as a chance to build up her repertoire of healing skills:

> *This allowed me to accept any failures because these failures never subtracted from my "getting better times." A failure did not mean all was lost. . . . I could not throw up next time. At those times I would use the failures to examine the circumstances that led me to throw up. From this, I could learn to avoid certain circumstances. At first I thought this was weak, that I should be able to face anything to really be getting better. But I also had to face that I needed to build up my repertoire of holding in food, so I could get stronger, and if that meant playing games with myself, that was okay. I became more self-accepting, which enabled me to feel better about myself. I began to carefully examine how I felt after I had thrown up and also how I felt when I didn't. I gained greater trust in myself and in my ability to get well if I chose to.*

I found the same depth of self-forgiveness among the winners I interviewed who'd beaten Binge-Eating Fat. One woman offered this encouragement: "You have to realize you'll backslide at times. That's okay. It's part of the healing: two steps forward, one back. Just forgive yourself and go on. If you allow yourself to flare up without guilt, you'll short-circuit anxiety and be less likely to binge. When you fall off the wagon, just take that as a sign you're not 'perfect' yet. Welcome to the human race!"

8. Trust in God

Winners who beat Binge-Eating Fat are also often deeply motivated and inspired by their faith. In a survey of 217 recovered and recovering binge eaters by Hall and Cohn, 42 percent mentioned spirituality as one of their "treatments" that worked. Hall and Cohn note, "The specific religions and practices varied." Mentioned were worshiping God or Jesus Christ or following their guru; doing zazen; or embracing Buddhism. Self-love and love for other people also had spiritual effects with the same positive consequences.

Women talked about "practicing love instead of self-pity" and "facing fears instead of running from them." One winner said: "The main thing that has helped me is my faith and trust in God. A lack of security is a problem with eating disorder sufferers, and knowing God cares for me gives me comfort and peace. We all need someone to trust [who] we know loves us unconditionally, not for how we look or what we do, just for us as we are."

Many binge-eating winners believe deeply in God's healing, a belief that's now repeatedly being supported by hard science. Even when people don't know they're being prayed for, they often recover. Rudy, a binge eater for six years, had "done everything," exhausting all her options. One day, a friend put her name on the prayer list at her local church. Each week, a group of devout parishioners prayed for Rudy to "find the wisdom to solve her own problem." Slowly, Rudy began to recover. She's been binge-free for three years.

Where to Go Next

Once you've broken your binge patterns, if you still need to lose weight, go to Chapter 19, "Designing Your Superconfidence Diet."

For more ways to cope with stress, see Chapter 9, "Losing Daily Hassles Fat."

If you go into a trance or "numb out" when you eat, go to Chapter 18, "Losing Post-Trauma Fat."

If you eat mostly at night, also check out Chapter 15, "Losing Night-Eating Fat."

Since Binge-Eating Fat often goes hand in hand with depression, see Chapter 10, "Losing Depression Fat," for ways to lift your moods.

CHAPTER 14

Losing Polycystic Ovary Fat

Internal balance is health, and internal unbalance is sickness.

—Clarence Cook Little, M.D.

For Angela, a twenty-seven-year-old preschool teacher in Jefferson City, Missouri, the nightmare began at puberty. She says, "I was chubby as a child, so my mom and stepdad (both fat themselves) had always badgered me to slim down. But after I started my periods at age twelve, I just kept getting fatter, no matter how little I ate or how much I exercised. I tried Weight Watchers, liquid fasts, Jenny Craig, no-fat, low-fat, all-pasta, you name it. Nothing worked."

When Angela was thirteen, she saw a behavioral psychologist, who devised a new form of torture. "He put me on what he called his 'reward' diet, but what I secretly called the Diet From Hell. Every Friday after school, I had to go to his office and weigh in. If I'd failed to lose weight, he ridiculed me for being ugly, and I had to give him five dollars. If I lost weight, he was supposed to praise me and give me five dollars, but that rarely happened." Hence, from a tender age, Angela learned an oppressive societal message commonly sent to overweight women: "Because you're fat, you're ugly and you don't deserve anything, including respect or money." She sighs, "I also learned that no matter how diligently I tried, my hard work would always go unrewarded."

After Angela became sexually active at seventeen and went on the birth-control pill, her weight went completely out of control. Each year from then on, she gained 20 pounds. "By the time I was twenty-two, married, and wanted a baby, I weighed 245. When we couldn't get pregnant, my husband, Bill, and I started down the primrose path of infertility treatment. Five doctors said I was too fat to conceive. They all told me to eat less and exercise more (like I haven't heard *that* before!). I was devastated. For a while, I ate one granola bar for breakfast, one granola bar for lunch and a 'sensible' dinner (no meat). In three months, I lost only three pounds." When she told one doctor how few calories she ate, he just rolled his eyes toward the ceiling in disbelief.

"Finally, a sixth doctor looked at my blood tests, did an ultrasound, and told me I had PCOS. I asked, 'What the hell's that?' He explained that it was an infertility disease caused by being overweight."

In fact, Angela's doctor was wrong on two counts. First, PCOS, or Polycystic Ovary Syndrome, is not an "infertility disease." It's a complex metabolic disorder that, if left untreated, can lead to a multitude of health problems, including not only infertility but also heart disease, diabetes, and endometrial cancer. Second, extra weight is a *symptom* of PCOS, not the *cause*.

Rather than treating her PCOS, the doctor simply put her on Clomid, a popularly prescribed infertility pill. When she returned for her fifth monthly office visit and still hadn't ovulated, he impatiently snapped, "Go home, and don't come back until you've lost 100 pounds." He blamed *her* because his treatment had failed.

Yet, sadly, by this time Angela had been so emotionally battered for her weight, she shouldered the blame. "I thought it was all my fault, and we'd never have a family just because I was fat. Bill tried to console me. But I cried all the way home."

Convinced she was "too fat to be a mother," she became deeply depressed. She enviously hated any pregnant woman she saw. Two years later, after consulting a total of seven physicians, she still hadn't been correctly treated for PCOS, she was still infertile, and she now weighed 298 pounds.

In her nightmarish struggles, Angela wasn't nearly as alone as she felt. An estimated 8 to 10 percent of women in North America and Europe have PCOS, although the vast majority don't know it. Between 50 and 80 percent of PCOS sufferers are overweight.

Is This Your Problem?

1. Do you have irregular, painful, or nonexistent periods? Did you start menstruating late?

2. Are you infertile?
3. Do men in your family tend to get bald in their twenties or thirties?
4. Do you struggle with thick, coarse hair on your face, arms, back, or tummy (from your pubic region up to your navel)?
5. Do you have female relatives on either your father's or mother's side who have any of these symptoms?
6. Has a doctor ever said you have cysts on your ovaries?
7. Do some women in your family, whatever their weight, have very thin, wispy hair on their heads?
8. Do you have brown, velvety patches of skin on the back of your neck?
9. Do you have oily skin or acne?
10. Do early heart disease, diabetes, and/or endometrial cancer run in your family?

If you answered yes to several of these questions, you need to find an endocrinologist who understands PCOS and get tested.

The Many Faces of PCOS

No two PCOS sufferers are exactly alike. Some struggle with oily skin and acne. Others have peaches-and-cream complexions. Some have embarrassing facial hair, so thick and coarse they have to shave their chins and upper lips or curl their "sideburns." Others have so little hair on their heads they fear they might become bald. Some are infertile. Others have three or four children before the full-blown syndrome erupts.

Yet despite this diversity, if you have Polycystic Ovary Fat, you'll share one common complaint with other sufferers. You'll have, in one winner's words "a hell of a time losing weight." The standard "eat less, exercise more" formula seldom works for you. Even if you heroically manage to shed a few pounds, you soon gain them all back.

In some cases, PCOS weight accumulates slowly but relentlessly, starting in adolescence. But in other cases, it piles on shockingly fast. Shortly after she went off the birth-control pill at age twenty-nine, one Pittsburgh woman with undiagnosed PCOS gained 100 pounds in less than six months. The good news: if you have this disorder, once you get your hormones in balance, you should have a much easier time slimming down.

The First Step Toward Healing: Learning the Facts

Originally called Stein-Leventhal Syndrome after the two doctors who first described it in 1935, *Polycystic Ovary Syndrome* takes its present name from the distinctive pearly-white cysts dotting many affected women's ovaries. Since doctors now know some PCOS patients don't have these cysts, however, the syndrome's name may change once again.

There are two types of PCOS: "thin" (the kind normal-weight women have); and "fat" (which goes hand in hand with being overweight). One frustrating symptom of the latter is unwanted body hair, found in 60 percent of overweight women. This bothersome hair can grow anywhere, but most frequently appears on your tummy, inner thighs, breasts, back, chin, forearms, legs, upper lip, or outer cheeks. The more overweight you are, the more likely you are to have this problem.

Though PCOS may be triggered by severe stress, it may also have a strong genetic component. (This is one condition in which genes *and* environment may both play a role.) In one study of sixty-one British families in which PCOS had been diagnosed, forty-five out of fifty-two sisters were afflicted with the disorder. Compared to women with "thin" PCOS, those with fat PCOS tend to have been heavier at birth and born to overweight mothers, a finding suggesting that your extra weight may have begun in the womb. A history of diabetes, endometrial cancer, high cholesterol, and early heart disease (before age sixty among the women in your family) can be another tip-off that you could either have this disorder or be vulnerable to it.

Also, look at the men in your family. Are any of them prematurely bald? Two studies published in *Clinical Endocrinology* suggest one gene that promotes PCOS in women may also cause premature baldness in men. Men in PCOS families also tend to be overweight and at higher risk for heart attacks.

A susceptibility to PCOS can be passed along by either parent. But you're more likely to develop this malady if PCOS runs in your dad's family. In one survey, 87 percent of females with PCOS on their father's side versus 47 percent with PCOS on their mother's side developed this metabolic imbalance. So look at your father's sisters or mother to see if they also struggled with weight, wispy hair, or other symptoms.

THE TESTOSTERONE FACTOR

Many blood abnormalities accompany PCOS, but the one linked closest to visceral fat is having too many male sex hormones (called *androgens*). There are several types of androgens, but the most potent is testosterone. If your hormones are properly balanced, your body contains about one-fortieth the amount of testosterone found in the average man; but if you have fat PCOS, you may have ten times that amount. At University College and Middlesex School of Medicine in London, a team of endocrinologists led by Dr. Gerald S. Conway carefully measured many different hormones in women with PCOS. Only testosterone accompanied higher body weights. Women with the highest testosterone levels also weighed the most. Because this hormone selectively stores more fat in your abdomen (the pattern more typical of men), having PCOS practically guarantees you'll have higher-than-normal amounts of unhealthy visceral fat. The prime villain causing all the other metabolic problems associated with PCOS, however, appears to be high insulin levels.

ASSOCIATED HEALTH PROBLEMS

Many overweight PCOS sufferers also have other signs of the Deadly Quartet, including a failure to use insulin efficiently. As a result, when you're struggling with this way to be fat, you need to get your blood pressure, trigylcerides, HDL and LDL cholesterol, and insulin or blood sugar levels checked regularly. Adult-onset diabetes typically doesn't strike women until their fifties or sixties; but if you have PCOS, you can get diabetes in your twenties or thirties. PCOS also raises the risk of early heart disease. A Swedish study found that women in their forties or fifties with PCOS were *seven times* more likely to suffer heart attacks than those the same age without PCOS. Translation: having PCOS (if it's ignored and untreated) can put you as much at risk for a heart attack as smoking three packs of cigarettes a day. If you go months without a period, the buildup of tissue in your uterine lining may also increase your risk of endometrial cancer.

Fortunately, if PCOS is caught early (the sooner the better), a healthy diet and exercise coupled with new medical treatments and stress reduction can prevent most, if not all, these associated health problems. So in a way, Polycystic Ovary Fat is simply a yellow flag warning you to nurture your body's needs before more serious problems develop.

Getting an Accurate Diagnosis

Full-blown cases of this syndrome are easy to spot, especially if you're overweight and have lots of body hair. Early stages of this condition, however, can be easily missed. To get an accurate diagnosis, your best bet is to visit an endocrinologist at a university weight-loss clinic. In addition to the standard cholesterol, insulin action, and blood pressure tests for the Deadly Quartet described in Chapter 7, your doctor also needs to order blood tests that measure your levels of male sex hormones. Total testosterone levels matter, but according to Andrea Dunaif, M.D., a PCOS researcher at Brigham and Women's Hospital in Boston, the most sensitive test for PCOS is the one that measures your free testosterone levels. So be sure to ask your doctor for that one. A third male hormone—DHEA-S—should also be measured.

When getting your hormones tested, time of day also counts. Hormone levels rise and fall throughout the day, and testosterone tends to be lowest in midafternoon. So schedule your blood work for the morning. If you're convinced you have PCOS but your tests come back normal, you may want to get retested.

What about getting a pelvic ultrasound to see if you have cysts on your ovaries? This diagnostic test is commonly ordered in Europe, but not in the United States. Why the difference? The controversy springs from the fact that an ultrasound alone isn't enough to confirm PCOS. Before menopause, between 22 and 33 percent of women have ovaries that *appear* polycystic, but only about 10 percent of women actually have the full-blown syndrome. Still, if your male hormones are high and an ultrasound shows your ovaries are also enlarged and dotted with pearly cysts, the diagnosis is confirmed. It's not any single test but the combination of several tests, along with detailed personal and family histories, that provide a definitive diagnosis.

Exploring Options, Making Choices

No single treatment is right for all women. The secret is to work with your doctor to explore the pros and cons of each approach, then choose the best plan for you. With this goal in mind, here are three key questions to ponder:

1. WHAT HAS YOUR EXPERIENCE BEEN WITH THE PILL?

Did you gain—or lose—weight on it? Which pill were you on? While taking it, how healthy were your cholesterol, blood sugar, and blood pressure readings? Depending on their hormonal formulas, different birth-control pills can affect your hormones and weight differently.

Some birth-control pills can help you lose weight. In one University of Gothenburg study, women with PCOS went on birth-control pills for eight months. *All* of those women who'd been 20 percent or more over their ideal weights when the study began lost 10 to 20 percent of their body weight. For a 200-pound woman, that's 20 to 40 pounds. As an added benefit, the pill can slow the growth of unwanted body hair and regulate your periods, thereby reducing your risk for endometrial cancer.

If you want to try the pill to rebalance your hormones and lose weight, just remember two things.

First, every woman's body responds to the pill differently. When one woman with thin PCOS went on the pill, she *gained* 26 pounds. Trust your body's signals, and don't view this treatment as a panacea.

Second, if you do take the pill, make sure your doctor prescribes a brand containing progestins with almost no androgen activity. Some of the older pills contain progestins (artificial forms of the hormone progesterone) that act like androgens in the body. Since your weight is linked to the fact that you *already* have too many androgens in your blood, you don't want to aggravate your problems by adding more. Four low-androgen pills that won't increase your testosterone are OrthoCyclen, Ortho Trycyclen, OrthoCept, and Desogen. Older formula pills you'll want to avoid contain *norgestrel* or *norethindrone*, two progestins that frequently cause weight gain and acne.

Another PCOS treatment you'll want to avoid is cyproterone acetate (CPA), the drug most frequently prescribed in Europe to get rid of excess hair. Sold under the brand name Androcur, this medication has been likened to a "superstrong birth-control pill." Its most common side effects are fatigue, loss of libido, and—once again—*weight gain*. It's not available in the United States, so I mention it only for anyone getting treatment in Europe. Spironolactone is commonly prescribed with the pill to get rid of unwanted body hair. But you shouldn't take spironolactone if you're trying to get pregnant.

2. How Do You Feel about Taking Medications?

You should never take pills until you know their possible side effects and have weighed all the risks. Even aspirin can damage your gastrointestinal tract if you take it too often. Still, if other treatments fail to help you balance your hormones and lose weight, a diabetes medication called metformin (sold under the brand name Glucophage) could be just what the doctor ordered. Available for years in Canada and Europe and FDA-approved in 1995 in the United States as a treatment for Type II diabetes, metformin corrects many of the blood abnormalities associated with PCOS. It can reduce high insulin levels, lower triglycerides, fight "bad" LDL cholesterol, raise "good" HDL cholesterol, lower testosterone, get rid of acne, reduce facial hair—and help you lose weight.

Several years ago, a team of more than one hundred physicians across the country conducted a controlled, double-blind study of metformin on over one thousand people with Type II diabetes. The study was headed by Ralph A. DeFronzo, M.D., at the University of Texas Health Science Center in San Antonio and reported in the *New England Journal of Medicine*. One group taking metformin lost an average of 8 or 9 pounds without formally dieting. The weight loss was only about one-third of a pound a week. But it was *steady*.

A number of smaller studies of PCOS patients have also verified that metformin promotes weight loss. Dr. Charles Glueck of Jewish Hospital/Alliance Hospitals Cholesterol Center in Cincinnati found in one study that when women with PCOS took metformin for eight weeks, their body mass indexes (BMIs) were reduced by 1.3 percent. For a 200-pound woman, that's a loss of about 12 pounds in eight weeks—not bad. But the news gets even better: Dr. Glueck reports that among his patients, some women who stay on metformin *continue* to lose. "The result can be very dramatic," he says. "A few women lose 50, 60, or 70 pounds." Unfortunately, some of this weight loss may be due to the fact that this drug makes many women nauseous.

Metformin can also lead to an extremely rare but potentially deadly toxic buildup of lactic acid in the blood, called lactic acidosis. Metformin normally passes unmetabolized through your body and is then secreted in your urine. But if your kidneys malfunction for any reason, metformin can build up rapidly and lactic acidosis can result. Metformin doesn't *cause* your kidneys to stop working. It only leads to lactic acidosis if they do.

How likely is this problem? Statistically, if one hundred thousand women with PCOS took metformin for a year, three would develop lactic acidosis. If ten million took it for two years, six hundred would develop it. Since you're an individual, not a statistic, seek out a competent doctor, ask plenty of questions, and stay alert for new treatments. Several newer medications in development at this writing, including an insulin-sensitizing drug called D-chiro-inositöl, may be better for you.

3. Are You Comfortable Experimenting with Herbs?

Manindri, thirty, a petite housewife with PCOS from North Carolina, reports that Chinese herbs gave her more energy, helped rebalance her hormones, and also helped her go from 145 to 112 pounds. Other PCOS sufferers also report great successes with herbs.

Will herbs also work for you? You won't find this question answered in any Western medical journal. But since Chinese herbal therapy seeks to rebalance the whole body—and since the key defining characteristic of PCOS is that it throws your whole system out of whack—herbs may be worth trying. One drawback to herbs: since they're not FDA-approved, some herbs fail to contain the ingredients listed on the labels or contain unlisted ingredients. A product labeled "natural" can still have unsafe side effects. In case of doubt, seek the help of an open-minded physician, or a skilled Chinese herbalist. Here are two herbs you may want to explore:

Fructus lycii. Also known under the Chinese name *gou qi zi*, this herb, actually a sweet Chinese berry, is said to be especially good for rebalancing the whole reproductive system, both the ovaries and the uterus in women and the testicles and prostate in men. Western herbalists and naturopaths prescribe it to enhance fertility, soften skin, relieve fatigue, and regulate blood sugar—all types of healing many PCOS sufferers could use.

I found no published studies in which *lycii* was tested to help women with PCOS lose weight. But several studies have linked this herb to some of the blood abnormalities common in PCOS. Overweight women with PCOS, for example, frequently have high levels of cholesterol and triglycerides. One study of 130 people done in Shenyang and reported in the *Journal of Traditional Chinese Medicine* found that a combination of herbs (one of which was *Fructus lycii*) worked remarkably well for these problems. It lowered cholesterol in 87 percent of cases and triglycerides in 81 percent. Another study done at Sun Yat-Sen University of Medical Sciences found some substances in *Fructus lycii* "protected" DNA in such a way that this herb may "play an important role in preventing cancer," researchers noted. *Fructus lycii* certainly hasn't been proved effective by Western scientific standards. That will probably never happen unless a pharmaceutical company with deep pockets decides to invest. But if you'd like to try it, dried berries are available by mail order. You can find sources on the Internet. *Lycii* berries are also available in Chinese grocery stores and can be eaten fresh or tossed into fruit salads or muffins.

Dong quai. Dong quai (*Angelica sinesis*) is best known in this country as one of several herbal remedies for perimenopausal hot flashes. Among Chinese medicine practitioners, it's known as "the sovereign herb for women" because of its power to regulate menstrual cycles and "strengthen the womb." It's also used to treat abdominal pain, menstrual cramps, and heart disease, all problems common in PCOS. Dong quai is considered one of the "tonic" herbs, meaning it will make your whole system more balanced, resilient, and disease-resistant. Andrew Weil, M.D., the well-known Harvard-educated expert on medicinal plants, suggests: "If you want to experiment with [dong quai], try taking two capsules of the root twice a day or one dropperful of the tincture in a little water twice a day. Give it a six-to-eight-week trial to see what it does for you." Dong quai shouldn't be used if you have problems with fibroids (which feed on estrogen) or excessive menstrual bleeding. Before taking this or any other herb for PCOS, talk to your health provider.

Other tips:

• If you have PCOS, be sure to share what you learn about it with everybody in your family. Even thin women and men without obvious symptoms may have hidden metabolic problems, such as poor insulin control or high blood pressure. Catching and controlling such problems early is the surest route to preventing heart disease, diabetes, stroke, and some cancers.

• If you think you once had Polycystic Ovary Fat but are now past menopause so your symptoms have subsided, be sure to continue getting regular medical checkups. In one study, women who recalled having PCOS-like symptoms when they were younger were more likely to have heart attacks in their sixties. As a good rule of thumb, get your blood pressure, cholesterol, and blood sugar checked regularly. If you still have your uterus, it's also wise to get screened annually for endometrial cancer.

• Winners who beat Polycystic Ovary Fat frequently report using a controlled-carbohydrate, high-protein, relatively high-fat diet like the one described in *Sugar Busters!* "It was the only weight-loss diet that ever worked for me," reports Jill, the winner you met in Chapter 8. Why? For one thing, a diet that's about 30 to 35 percent fat or maybe a little higher is often easier to stick with because it's tastier and more satisfying than a low-fat diet. A diet richer in fat also keeps your insulin levels in check. Insulin alone doesn't make you fat. But in the presence of insulin, cortisol causes you to store fat faster. So when you control your insulin levels, you at least *slow down* unhealthy fat storage. When you control your stress levels, of course, you lower your rate of unhealthy-fat storage even more. By keeping insulin levels in check, a controlled-carbohydrate diet also helps combat the other blood abnormalities that often accompany PCOS. When cutting out the "bad" carbs (mostly sugars, white flours, and starchy vegetables like potatoes), however, be sure not to skimp on the "good" carbs: fruits, nonstarchy vegetables, and whole grains. Good carbohydrates, from oranges to oatmeal, contain "phytochemicals" (literally "plant chemicals") that fight many illnesses, from heart disease to cancer.

When you have Polycystic Ovary Fat, it's also important to consider the *types* of fats you consume. A diet high in "bad" saturated animal fats like those in red meats, butter, cream, and cheeses appears to make PCOS worse, whereas a diet rich in "good" fats like those in nuts as well as canola and olive oils appears to improve this complex disorder. Still, you're an individual. Your best eating plan is the one that makes *you* the healthiest. Go to Chapter 19, "Designing Your Superconfidence Diet," for more information.

• Limit alcohol, switch from coffee and caffeinated sodas to herbal teas, and absolutely don't smoke. All these ersatz stress relievers can prolong or raise cortisol secretions, which in turn may be the first trigger leading to the cascade of metabolic disturbances that characterize this disorder.

• Try to exercise diligently. It may not help you lose much *weight*, but when you have PCOS, it's one of the best things you can do for your health, and it can do wonders to rebalance your hormones. Go to Chapter 20, "Becoming an Exercise Winner," for information every woman with PCOS should know about exercise and how to stick with it.

Since PCOS may be initially triggered by extreme stress and is also an inherently stressful condition, you may also want to read Chapter 9, "Losing Daily Hassles Fat," and possibly Chapter 18, "Losing Post-Trauma Fat." Many women with this disorder also have thyroid problems, so go to Chapter 11, "Losing Lazy Thyroid Fat," as well.

When working to lose PCOS fat, you have many options—from medications to diet. But now that you know you're dealing with an endocrine imbalance (not a "lack of willpower"), you'll be far more able to find the help you need and make choices that work.

CHAPTER 15

Losing Night-Eating Fat

We are not only what we eat, but when we eat.

—*Chronobiologist Franz Halberg*

You go to bed, only to toss and turn restlessly. You immediately know it will be one of "those" nights. You soon find yourself obsessing about those chocolate chip cookies in the cupboard. Maybe if you had just one, you could go to sleep. . . . You get up. Three cookies later, you're back in bed and fall asleep like a baby. Unfortunately, the bliss is short-lived. Two hours later, you're up once again, prowling through the kitchen, raiding the refrigerator for that piece of leftover peach pie. Before morning, you may get up several more times. Since all this eating takes place under cover of darkness, nobody knows about it but you.

If you eat this way, you may think you're all alone. In fact, you have a long-ignored disorder called Night-Eating Syndrome (NES). Although NES was first observed by Pennsylvania University's Albert Stunkard in 1955, it has only recently been recognized as a distinctly separate disorder. About 10 percent of overweight women who go to clinics and up to 27 percent of seriously overweight women struggle with this surprisingly common way to be fat.

Too little sleep can contribute to anybody's weight problems. Studies show that when you're sleep-deprived, you tend to eat more. But the *amount* of sleep isn't all that matters; *quality* also counts. In one study, when eight students were deprived of rapid eye movement (REM) sleep for several nights, five felt hungrier and three gained weight.

Although sleeping less may enable you to burn 10 to 15 percent more calories than usual during the day, sleep deprivation usually leads to an increased *consumption* of more than 10 to 15 percent as you try to boost your energy. Too little sleep may also cause you to lose body heat so you eat more in an effort to stay warm.

When you have NES, your stomach is probably queasy when you get up in the morning. Breakfast? *Blech!* The very thought makes you cringe. Even at lunch, you may eat very little. But as the day progresses, your hunger builds. From 4 P.M. on, your energy flags and your moods dip lower with each passing hour. As cortisol mounts, you feel stressed and depressed.

Once home, you start snacking. In one study conducted jointly by Stunkard's team and a group of endocrinologists in Norway, night eaters ate nine times during a twenty-four-hour period compared to four times for people without this condition. People with normal eating patterns consume about 75 percent of their calories before 6 P.M. and eat very little after 8 P.M. In comparison, you may take in less than 40 percent of your total calories by 6 P.M. and continue eating rapidly until after midnight. You may also wake up three or more times a night and consume more than half of your total calories after you go to bed.

Is this just a night-owl variation of binge eating? No. That's the surprising part. In fact, if you have NES, you probably *don't* binge. During a binge, people average a whopping 1,900 calories, and some eat 6,000 to 10,000 calories or more at a sitting. Night Eaters tend to eat only about 270 calories per snack.

Can you binge *and* night-eat? Sure. But if you do, you have two interconnected problems: binge fat and night eating fat. Your best way to win in this case might be to view your way to be fat as a nesting syndrome and attack each problem separately.

Is This Your Problem?

1. Do you have a total lack of appetite in the mornings, even if you force yourself to eat breakfast?
2. Do you consume 50 percent or more of your daily calories *after* your evening meal?
3. Do you wake up at least once a night and sometimes eat during those times?

4. Have you been struggling with insomnia and middle-of-the-night eating for three months or longer?
5. Do you *not* meet the criteria for Binge-Eating Syndrome?

If you answered yes to all these questions, you may have Night-Eating Syndrome.

The Body Clock Connection

Since NES is only beginning to be studied, the exact causes remain cloudy. But certainly stress plays a role. Stunkard reports overweight women's night eating intensifies during high-stress periods and lessens when they relax. Depression may be involved, too.

The key problem underlying all NES symptoms, however, appears to be an out-of-whack body clock. Approximately every twenty-four hours, your hormones rise and fall in predictable cycles known as circadian rhythms. These cycles are "reset" every day, mostly by your exposure to light and by regular habits such as the times you eat or exercise. When your circadian rhythms get thrown off balance (as they do when you suffer jet lag, for example), many side effects can erupt, including fatigue, depression, frazzled nerves, fragmented sleeping patterns, and imbalanced eating patterns.

Though we often fail to realize it, eating and sleeping are part of the same daily rhythm. Like ocean waves, your daily rhythms continually rise and fall, inextricably interconnected. If you're eating poorly, you may also be sleeping poorly, and vice versa. Robbed of a refreshing night's sleep, you may barely have enough energy to drag yourself through the day. When you're exhausted, your body also burns fewer calories and hoards fat, explains Stanford University sleep authority William C. Dement, author of *The Promise of Sleep*.

When you're struggling with NES, you very likely have many chemical imbalances other people don't have. You probably have elevated cortisol (indicating chronic stress) throughout the day. You may also have much lower-than-normal nighttime levels of leptin (which regulates hunger). In most people, leptin levels rise at night, suppressing appetite. With NES, leptin levels stay low, so you stay hungry.

Perhaps the most important hormone in this syndrome is melatonin, which induces sleep and resets the body's biological clock. According to Dement, "Melatonin is the hormone that seems to communicate the pulse of the biological clock to every cell in the body." With your melatonin thrown off, your body clock can't keep accurate time. Most people's melatonin levels rise right before bedtime and stay high through the night, only beginning to taper off around 4 A.M. In NES sufferers, melatonin is much lower than normal throughout the night. Result: you find it much harder to go to sleep, and you keep waking up.

Some women report their NES worsens right before their periods. If this happens, you may have what's called "premenstrual insomnia," a kind of bad case of jet lag without the frequent flier miles. During this sleep disturbance, melatonin is blunted throughout the day, and even bright light may not raise it. Sleep problems and night eating may worsen with age and during the hormonal swings of menopause. Shift work can also throw off your body clock's delicate timing and trigger or intensify night eating.

Surprising Ways to Sleep and Get Thin

In a very real way, NES may be a *sleep* problem as much as it is an eating disorder. As one sufferer put it: "If I could only sleep through the night, I wouldn't even be tempted to eat. I'd cut my calorie intake in half. Also, if I got a good night's rest, I'd have more energy during the day and feel more like exercising."

Since your biological clock can be reset both by proper eating and proper sleeping (the two are interconnected), here are fourteen great ways to reduce night eating and also get a slimming night's rest.

1. EAT THREE MEALS

Eat at *exactly the same hours* each day. "I'm never hungry for breakfast, but I realized that was part of my problem. So I forced myself to eat anyway," says Lauren, a thirty-seven-year-old Minneapolis attorney with NES who used to nibble almost constantly after she got home from work. "At first, looking at food in the morning turned my stomach. But, after a few weeks, I guess my clock got rewound, and I began getting hungry before breakfast. Now I eat three meals a day and have much more energy than I used to. I've also lost 22 pounds."

2. ELIMINATE SNACKS

"I realized I was probably confusing my body clock by eating at all sorts of odd times. So I stopped snacking—completely. That, coupled with learning how to get a good night's sleep, solved my night eating completely," " says Christie, a waitress from Lansing, Michigan, who lost 39 pounds of Night-Eating Fat.

3. EAT FAVORITE FOODS FOR BREAKFAST

If you deny yourself delectable treats all day, you may eat them at night anyway when you're tired and your defenses are down. Some women even sleepwalk in order to eat cookies, cake, and ice cream. The solution? Many winners report choosing the foods they love most for breakfast and save "boring" choices like carrots and cabbage for evening grazing. "Brie, crackers, and Kona coffee for breakfast?" one winner laughs. "Hey, it works for me!" (She reminds me of my grandmother who ate crackers and coffee as her "morning cereal," was slim all her life, and lived to be ninety-four.)

4. CUT THE CAFFEINE

Be especially careful about drinking caffeine after 6 P.M. Caffeine stays in your system for hours. Even if you drink only one cup of coffee, tea, or caffeinated cola for dinner, you could still have some caffeine left in your system at 11 P.M. What's more, the older you get, the more easily stimulants like caffeine may disrupt your sleep patterns. (Also beware of caffeine-containing pills like Midol.)

5. QUIT SMOKING

Smokers sleep more poorly than nonsmokers. Although nicotine withdrawal may disturb your sleep at first, you'll soon breathe better and sleep more soundly.

6. CHECK OUT YOUR MEDICATIONS

We'll review many drugs that can make you fat in Chapter 17. But some prescription and over-the-counter medications can also keep you awake—and possibly set the stage for night eating. Insomnia promoters include gastrointestinal drugs like Tagamet; heart and

blood-vessel medications like Inderol, HydroDURIL, and Meva-
cor; thyroid medications like Synthroid; nicotine gums or patches
designed to help you stop smoking; and cold, cough, allergy, or
asthma drugs like Sudafed. Paradoxically, *withdrawing* from some
asthma medications can also keep you awake. If you need a medication that's giving you insomnia (and thereby making you fat), ask
your doctor about changing the *timing* of your dosage. Often just
changing the time of day when you take medications will determine
whether you can sleep through the night.

7. GET OUTSIDE AT NOON

One winner noticed that if she took her brisk walk in the early-
morning sunshine instead of at 4:30 or 5 P.M., she ate less in the evening and also slept better. Does this make sense? Yes. Melatonin, the
body-clock hormone, is changed not only by the *amount* of daylight
you get, but also by *when* you get it. Lots of bright light early in the
morning will make you sleepy *earlier* in the evening. Bright light
later in the day makes you sleepy *later*. If you're having trouble falling asleep at night, sleep experts recommend avoiding all bright
light in late afternoon (if you have to go out, wear sunglasses).

8. WORK TO BEAT STRESS

NES intensifies under stress. So does insomnia. At least half of
insomniacs consider "the hyperarousal caused by stress and worry"
the main cause of their sleep problems. If you lie in bed fretting
about everything from your bills to tomorrow's deadlines, try setting aside a thirty-minute "worry time" several hours before bedtime, Dement suggests. During this half hour, you're required to *do
nothing but worry*. This works in a kind of paradoxical way; after a
while, worry becomes so tediously dull you either stop doing it or
start seeking solutions. See Chapter 9, "Losing Daily Hassles Fat,"
for many other ways to reduce stress.

9. AVOID LATE-NIGHT WORKOUTS

Although some robust souls can pump iron then drop right off to
sleep, most of us become so hyperalert after a workout we require
several hours to calm down. For your best chance of getting a good
night's rest, stop all exercise routines three hours before bedtime.
Will exercise alone help you sleep better? Eventually, maybe.

Studies have shown trained athletes spend more time in the deep, restful stages of sleep. If you've just started working out, though, you may sleep worse for a while, as stiff muscles keep you awake. If you do shift work, regular exercise may also help your circadian rhythms adapt faster to the new routine, especially if you also expose yourself to light at the right times of day (see number 7 on page 176).

10. KNOW YOUR LIMITS

Alcohol also has paradoxical effects on sleep. Half a glass of port or white wine before bedtime might make you sleep better. But too much alcohol disrupts sleep patterns, so you tend to wake up around 2 A.M. as the alcohol wears off. Recovering alcoholics have extremely disrupted sleep patterns and are often plagued with terrifying nightmares. This may explain why 75 percent of recovering alcoholic women in one study reported night eating. If you find yourself depending on alcohol to get to sleep, that's a sign you're headed for trouble.

11. WIND DOWN GENTLY

Try not to get excited, angry, or anxious right before bedtime. Also don't check your e-mail, pay bills, worry about your kid's D in math, or watch the nightly news, with all those cortisol-raising stories about murders, rapes, fatal plane crashes, and corruption. Instead, wind down before sleep with a warm bath, soft music, or a gentle book. As you dowse the light and close your eyes, envision a wild-flower meadow, a lovely vacation spot, or some other idyllic scene.

12. KICK OFF THE COVERS

Temperature may affect sleep as much as light does. "Cooler temperatures act like dark; warmer temperatures act like light," says Jay Dunlap, professor of biochemistry at Dartmouth Medical School. (No surprise to menopausal women who find it impossible to sleep through 2 A.M. hot flashes.) When you wake up in the middle of the night and feel hot, try kicking off the covers, moving to a cooler room, or flipping on the air conditioner.

13. AVOID BRIGHT LIGHTS AT NIGHT

Since light alters your melatonin levels and resets your body clock, keep lights dim in the evenings. Also, avoid staring at the computer screen right before bedtime. If you get up in the middle of the night, keep the lights low. Even a bright bathroom light at 2 A.M. can tell your body it's time to wake up (and start eating). If you need some illumination, buy a small night-light.

Could You Have Apnea?

A common disorder in which the sufferer repeatedly stops breathing for a few seconds to a minute or longer, obstructive sleep apnea afflicts more than fifty million people in the United States alone and often goes undiagnosed. If you have this problem, each time you stop breathing you have to wake up to breathe. The result: you may frequently come fully awake, get up to pee, then head for the fridge.

The most obvious symptom is loud snoring, often "like a jackhammer." Other signs include impaired thinking, irritability, depression, high blood pressure, morning headaches, and chronic fatigue. The more overweight you are, the greater the odds you have this disorder and need to be treated.

Fortunately, apnea can often be treated with what's called a continuous positive airway pressure (CPAP) machine. The CPAP gently blows air into the nose through a mask. Some people find the mask uncomfortable; others don't mind. If you can get used to the CPAP, you'll soon sleep through the night. Result: you'll stop night eating and enjoy a great surge of energy during the day. After going on this treatment, one woman was so energized she lost 58 pounds in six months.

Another promising new treatment involves inserting tiny needles into the airway tissue (often at the back of the tongue) and using precision-directed radio-frequency waves to shrink the tissue causing the problem. If you suspect you may have apnea and want to know more, contact the National Sleep Foundation (729 15th St., NW, 4th Floor, Washington, D.C. 20005) for a list of sleep disorder centers in the United States.

14. CONSIDER MELATONIN

Since as a night eater, you probably have abnormally low melatonin levels before bedtime, should you take those melatonin pills available in health food stores? They may be worth a shot. Ask your doctor. Dement says that in very low doses (up to 0.5 milligrams for the average adult), melatonin can shift your biological clock. Still, he cautions, melatonin is not FDA-regulated, so it's hard to know how much you're getting in any given formula. Also, the vast majority of popular claims about "melatonin miracles" being able to cure everything from aging to the common cold have never been backed by science.

If you do try melatonin, Dement suggests timing your dosage with the daylight. If you want to get sleepier *earlier* than usual, try taking melatonin right after sundown. If you want to fall asleep *later* and get up later, try taking it in the morning.

Where to Go Next

If you binge, be sure to review Chapter 13, "Losing Two Kinds of Binge-Eating Fat."

To reduce stress, go to Chapter 9, "Losing Daily Hassles Fat."

If you've ever been sexually molested or otherwise traumatized, read Chapter 18, "Losing Post-Trauma Fat." The hyperarousal that's keeping you awake in this case may spring from a deeper stress that you may need to address.

CHAPTER 16

Losing Post-Pregnancy Fat

Weight gain after childbirth is not solely a biological phenomenon.

—Lorraine O. Walker, R.N., Ed.D.
University of Texas at Austin
School of Nursing

To their disappointment, many women who've breezed along confident and thin for years suddenly find it impossible to slim down after a baby or two. You'll often hear that the "average" woman retains only four pounds after childbirth. If you've gained more, you may wonder where you've gone wrong. But statistical "averages" like this only undermine confidence and belie the actual experiences of many women.

In reality, post-pregnancy weights can fall anywhere on a wide continuum. In one Swedish study a year after delivery, some women had lost as many as 10 pounds over their pre-pregnancy weights. Others had gained more than 50 pounds. An estimated 40 to 50 percent of extremely overweight women say their pregnancies were an "important trigger" for their weight gains. That's when they put on lots of extra fat in a spurt.

We're often sold the idea that even after giving birth to three kids, we should still be able to run around the beach in our bikinis. It comes as a shock to many women when that's no longer an option. Alan Stein and coworkers at the Royal Free Hospital School of Medicine in London found that most new mothers are taken aback by how much weight they gained and how their body shape changed. Six months after delivery, 70 percent of new mothers are dissatisfied with the way their bodies look, and 39 percent are still unhappy a year later.

Having one baby, especially in your early twenties, may not change your body shape much. But having a second baby will often leave you a lot plumper and flabbier than you'd expected. Among women who started out at normal weights, pregnancy accounts for over half the weight gained during adulthood (aging accounts for the other half). C-sections, as you'll see in a minute, only add to the problem.

Is Post-Pregnancy Fat healthy? Some of it can be (if it's in the hips and thighs); but after pregnancy, many women also accumulate more fat in their visceral cells.

An Ounce of Prevention

Factors that can affect how much weight you'll retain after a pregnancy and how hard you'll struggle to lose it include your age, race, height (shorter women often stay fatter), genes, and the number of children you've had. But generally, the women most likely to stay overweight after childbirth are those who gained most while they were pregnant.

So how much should you gain to ensure a healthy baby without making yourself fat? Unfortunately, that's up for debate. About thirty years ago, when I was having babies, women were told to gain only about 20 to 25 pounds during pregnancy. The big medical fear in those days was toxemia (now called preeclampsia). If we restricted salt intake and watched our weight, we were reassured, we'd do just fine. I gained an average of 22 pounds with each of my pregnancies and gave birth to two perfectly healthy babies, both about 7 pounds.

Then the theory changed. The new idea became that if an underweight woman gained too little, she could have a low-weight baby with developmental problems, or even a stillborn. Suddenly, thin and normal-weight mothers were urged to gain 30 or even 40 pounds to protect their babies. Now the current guidelines are once again being disputed, as some experts argue they're making women too fat.

The current guidelines from the Institute of Medicine vary, depending on how much you weigh to start with. Here they are:

- Thin women (with BMIs of less than 19.8)—28 to 40 pounds

- Normal weight women (with BMIs of 19.8 to 26)—25 to 35 pounds
- Heavy women (with BMIs of 26 to 30)—15 to 25 pounds
- Obese women (with BMIs over 30)—15 pounds but not much more; too much increases risk to the baby.

So how many women in real life stick to these guidelines? Surprisingly few. Among two hundred pregnant women attending a clinic at St. Luke's–Roosevelt Hospital in New York City, 67 percent of the underweight women, 61 percent of the normal weight women, 69 percent of the overweight women, and 78 percent of the obese women did *not* follow the IOM guidelines. They either gained more or less than they "should have."

So if you still have time to prevent pregnancy fat, what does this mean to you? It means the amount you "should" gain to have a healthy baby is hardly set in stone. Blanket recommendations for all women may or may not apply to you as a unique individual. If you have concerns about gaining too much, talk to your doctor and ask lots of questions. You may find you can gain less than recommended and still have a happy, bouncy baby.

Once you've given birth and have already gained fat, you can lose it in any number of ways, depending on the underlying problem. But before we get to those, we need to discuss two common prescriptions that often don't work and can cause needless frustration.

The Exercise and Breast-Feeding Myths

You're often told you absolutely must exercise if you ever hope to get back into that little black dress. But, in fact, exercise may or may not help you regain your figure. One study found no relationship between exercise and weight loss in women six months after childbirth. In another finding from the University of Pennsylvania, the heaviest mothers were sometimes the ones who exercised *most*. (They also ate substantially no more calories than thin mothers did.) Exercise is certainly healthy, and it *may* work. It can reduce stress (a definite plus). But if it hasn't made your maternity fat disappear, you can rest assured you're not alone.

Another popular myth has it that breast-feeding will help you regain your figure faster than bottle-feeding. The truth: maybe so, maybe not. Whereas some breast-feeding moms do lose weight quickly, others *gain* fat, especially in the thighs and hips. You do burn more calories when you breast-feed. But whether this will reduce your weight is anybody's guess. Several studies even found that women who *bottle-fed* lost more weight and lost it faster. Breast milk can be very healthy for your baby, but choosing this method merely in hopes of losing weight may lead to disappointment.

Winning Ways to Beat Post-Pregnancy Fat

The outward changes in your life are obvious after having a baby. But much post-pregnancy distress—and distress fat—spring from the fact that you're also rapidly changing in many *unseen* ways. Your hormones are shifting (again!). Your body is regaining its balance after the miracle of giving birth. Your identity is broadening as you see yourself in a new light as a mother. You may have cut back or added to your workload. Your relationship with your husband and even your own parents may be changing for better or worse.

As you're going through this time of rapid change, here's how to take charge of your weight and keep it from spiraling out of control.

1. GO WITH THE FLOW

One insight that can help reduce stress-eating immensely during this time is realizing that growth (and confidence) proceed two steps forward and one step back. The new thinking teaches us it's okay to love being a mother one day and wish you could escape to a private island the next. It's normal to feel your life is better than ever and *almost at the same moment* to feel your whole world is falling apart. Such swings don't mean you're crazy. They're a normal, natural part of human growth at its best.

The unseen patterns of growth in your own life take place much as your baby grew in your womb. First, the growth was so slow it was barely noticeable. Slowly, the changes were more obvious. Then a sudden burst occurred as the baby came into the world. Your life is changing in much the same way. Human growth seldom proceeds as a smooth, steady, step-by-step process. Instead, we often build up slowly, then suddenly leap ahead in a burst, almost in a quantum leap of strength and awareness. This natural process of falling apart, then putting yourself back together again in new, more interesting ways is called resilience. It's a major hallmark of growth. But before you can make that quantum leap to a new level of maturity that's simultaneously freer and more responsible, you often experience a lot of stress. You may feel as if you're out of control because in many ways you *are* out of control. Reintegration in our lives is often preceded by a natural period of disintegration, as we break apart our old identities and cast aside those bits and pieces of ourselves that no longer work.

So how do you maintain your sanity in the midst of such turmoil? Try to relax. Embrace the change. Go with the flow. Reassure yourself that even if life feels very chaotic and disjointed right now, everything's as it should be. You (and if you're married, your husband) are simply in the process of incorporating a new baby into your much broader, much more interesting life. Will you and he fight more? Maybe. But these new power struggles, even if they feel awful at the time, can also be a sign of healthy growth, if you'll just hang in there. Over time, as you integrate this new little person into your family, the chaos will dwindle, order will reemerge, and you'll become calmer. That's when you'll find it much easier to lose weight.

One winner (now back to her pre-pregnancy weight) explains how this process worked in her life: "I was really struggling to get a grip after the second baby arrived. Trying to juggle a career with 3 A.M. feedings, getting my toddler off to preschool, and spending time with my husband was a real nightmare. Friends kept saying, 'You're so lucky, you've got it all,' and I'm thinking, 'Yeah, right, you try this sometime and see if you don't go nuts.' Before I could even begin to lose weight, I had to center myself." How? "I finally learned how to think of myself as the calm eye in the center of the hurricane. I've learned to step back from all the ruckus and hubbub, to separate myself emotionally from all the demands. I'll admit I had a good role model. My mother could always stay very centered and loving in the middle of all sorts of crises. Now I know what she was doing, how she did it. I've learned how to quietly watch all the chaos swirling around me: the dog's barking, the baby's crying, the phone's ringing—but inside I'm perfectly calm." Now *that's* super-confidence. (For tips on how to achieve this state yourself, go to Chapter 9, "Losing Daily Hassles Fat." See also "Observe Your Thoughts" on page 94.)

2. Smooth Out Your Rhythms

When a new baby comes into the house, everyone's rhythms are thrown out of whack. Eating, sleeping, and waking-up times can all become quite chaotic. When your rhythms are off, you feel lousy. At such times it's easy to gain weight and often hard to lose it. So try to get your rhythms back in sync by sticking as much as you can to a regular schedule. Even taking a fifteen-minute walk at the same time every day can help your circadian rhythms become smoother.

Katie, a neonatal nurse, is quite aware of a baby's need to establish rhythms. So she was also keenly conscious of her own rhythms as she worked to get back in shape. "As I worked to integrate the baby into our lives, I did lots of what I call 'rhythm work.' I did lots of rhythmic stretching. I listened to music and a tape of ocean waves. I tuned in to my own breathing while rocking the baby. I avoided alcohol altogether (even half a glass of white wine before bedtime can throw my sleep patterns off). I also tried to eat three small, regular meals a day, even if my husband, Jim, was working late. Rather than straining hard to do everything all at once, I tried to be gentle with myself, as gentle and patient as I am with my baby." As Katie's rhythms became less jangled, her eating patterns became less jangled. Six months after her baby was born, she was back to her pre-pregnancy weight.

3. Check Out Your Thyroid

If you were losing weight easily after the baby was born and then suddenly began gaining again, your thyroid (which plays a key role in metabolism) may be out of whack. About one in twenty women, maybe more, will develop what's called "postpartum thyroiditis." Since this condition typically occurs two to six months after delivery (some time after your last postpartum visit), it's frequently overlooked.

Symptoms are hard to distinguish from ordinary problems common among new mothers. The disorder usually starts with fatigue, irritability, and weight loss (all signs of an *over*active thyroid), then switches three to eight months after delivery to fatigue, constipation, and weight gain (all signs of an *under*active thyroid, also known as *hypothyroidism*). Dry skin, being oversensitive to cold, depression, mood swings, and even carpal tunnel syndrome have also been associated with this second, weight-gain phase of the disorder.

Why would your thyroid choose this particular time to go haywire? Because during pregnancy, your thyroid gland undergoes many changes, with the concentrations of some thyroid secretions rising as much as 200 to 300 percent. Although these changes are part of a normal pregnancy, after childbirth it can still take your system a while to calm down.

Tests to diagnose postpartum thyroiditis are the same as those used to diagnose other thyroid disorders, all of which are discussed in Chapter 11. The good news is that this condition will often straighten out on its own in a few months without treatment. Still, your doctor should follow you carefully, because a full-blown case of hypothyroidism develops in about 25 to 30 percent of cases. You should also have your thyroid tested during future pregnancies, since 10 to 25 percent of women who have thyroiditis during one pregnancy will get it again.

Anything else you can do? Yes. Don't pressure yourself to lose weight until your hormones settle down, and try to relax. Stress has also been strongly linked to thyroid disorders. Try to take this condition in stride, trusting that with time, your body will just naturally straighten itself out. Even if the problem persists, it can still be treated. Go to Chapter 11, "Losing Lazy Thyroid Fat," for more information.

4. REPLACE WORRY WITH PATIENCE

We're often taught it's good to feel unhappy with our weight, because that will "motivate" us to slim down faster. Yet, ironically, fretting over your weight too soon after childbirth can *prolong* your weight problems. In one British study, women who were most dissatisfied with their bodies after pregnancy had greater long-term weight *gains* than those who took their bodies' changes more in stride. In another British study, a few women who were extremely distressed about their weight after pregnancy developed full-blown eating disorders.

Stories of celebrity moms getting back in shape in just a few weeks only leave us frustrated and impatient. When we hear that supermodel Kim Alexis was out training for a 10K race three weeks after giving birth to her third child, we think, "If she can do it, why can't I?" But the truth is, we never hear about those celebrity moms who *fail* to achieve such apocryphal comebacks. In truth, only 28 percent of women in one study had returned to their pre-pregnancy weights six weeks after delivery. With patience, it's possible to get back in shape; but these things take time.

Weight worries are also heightened, because we're seldom told how much our bodies will change after a pregnancy. When we're confronted with flabbier abdominal muscles and wider hips than we ever expected (in other words, when we look more maternal), we're astonished. In her book *Operating Instructions*, Anne Lamott writes, "People kept trying to prepare me for how soft and mushy my stomach would be after I gave birth, but I secretly thought, Not this old buckarina. Oh, but now . . . when I lie on my side in bed, my stomach lies politely beside me, like a puppy."

The idea that we could lose weight calmly—without worry—goes counter to all popular belief. But winners have mastered this skill, mostly by making peace with a few extra pounds and focusing surprisingly little on food. Debra, who lost 32 pounds of Post-Pregnancy Fat after giving birth to twin boys, says: "Diets teach you to think constantly about food: what you'll eat, what you won't eat, good foods, bad foods. I'm convinced this is a terrible mistake. When I thought constantly about food, I just ate more and got fatter. When I thought about something else, most of the fat went away."

Many winners talk about filling their lives with so many interests they have no time to snack. Says one at-home mom: "Whenever I start to think about food, I cuddle my baby, study medieval art (my current passion), play with my cats, arrange flowers, or noodle around on the computer. I make myself too busy to eat." If you've become so worried about your weight that you're already on the dieting roller coaster, go to Chapter 13, "Losing Two Kinds of Binge-Eating Fat."

5. Enlist Help for Your Second Shift

A Duke University study suggests it's not being employed per se but working double time (what Arlie Hochschild called "the second shift") that leads to post-pregnancy weight gains. Working women with children at home had higher cortisol levels throughout the day than working women without children. What's more, the working moms' cortisol levels were highest at night, when many women are tempted to snack. This high-cortisol effect (which, as you now know, promotes visceral fat storage) occurred whether or not the women were married, no matter how much they earned or how high they'd scaled the corporate ladder, and no matter how supportive their husbands were.

Why? Part of it's simply the extra work, particularly for women. Total workload (which involves paid and unpaid work, including child care) increases directly with the number of children at home for both men and women. But women shoulder the bigger chunk of this burden: an employed mother's workload, on average, is two to three times higher than a father's.

So what's the answer? Turn over more chores to Dad? Yes, but it's more subtle than that. Kathleen C. Light, a psychologist at the University of North Carolina School of Medicine in Chapel Hill, suggests that although many women have already turned over household chores to their mates, they still haven't turned over the *vigilance* for getting those chores done. As a result, Light notes that "even when her partner is taking on more chores at home, the responsibility for seeing that the work gets done remains hers. Her sense of vigilance and being on call is virtually constant, whereas her spouse more often does his assigned chores and then relaxes." Studies have shown that fathers' effort hormones go down when they leave the office and head for home, whereas women's effort hormones at that point go *up*.

Even though many of us feel we've become liberated, the Superwoman Syndrome remains. Nearly half the women in a survey published in *Working Mother* said they felt stressed regularly, yet a whopping 60 percent said they simply shouldered the burdens by organizing themselves better and working harder. Only a scant 11 percent asked for extra help. "This pattern of remaining vigilant, responsible, and ready to work even harder struck a common chord with our research," Light notes. Women who embrace or even prefer "high-effort coping," tend to have elevated heart rates and blood pressures. Once they work themselves to exhaustion, their cortisol levels also soar.

If overwork is making you fat, give up more control. Ask your spouse to take on not just certain chores, but also the *responsibility* for getting those jobs done. Then kick back and relax. If it's his job to pay the electric bill or iron the kids' shirts and the electricity gets turned off or the kids go to school rumpled, that's *his* problem. Do you think you could never do that? Okay, look at it this way: you can give up control, relax, and get thin. Or you can stay in charge, stay tense, and stay fat. Go to Chapter 9, "Losing Daily Hassles Fat," for more tips on reducing your daily stress levels.

6. EXPLORE THOSE MATERNITY BLUES

Another often unaddressed cause of weight gain after childbirth is postpartum depression. If you're depressed, you're nearly twice as likely to gain 10 or more pounds as a happier new mom is.

What causes maternity blues? A lazy thyroid may be to blame, so rule that out first (see number 3 on page 185). High cortisol levels are another factor. Women who develop the blues have significantly higher cortisol levels than nonblues groups. What triggers high cortisol after pregnancy? Many factors can do it. But a major one is feeling unsupported by a spouse, family, or friends. Even a year after childbirth, feeling unsupported is related to depression, higher weight gains, and higher total body weight. Feeling unsupported, in turn, can lead to the high cortisol levels that are a hallmark of depression.

Women were once thought to succumb to the blues because they were somehow "disappointed" in their babies. But the issue is much more complex than that. Many women were depressed *before* the baby was born. In an Australian study, researchers found, "the most powerful predictor of the blues was a sense of 'pessimism' in late pregnancy, which was actually fulfilled by postpartum reality." Many women who suffered maternity blues reported that the pregnancy was unplanned and they'd considered abortions.

Childbirth can also reawaken conflicts with your own mother, triggering the doldrums. Lisa, who gained nearly 30 pounds during her postpartum depression, recalls, "When my daughter was born, it suddenly hit me how little I'd been nurtured as a little girl. On the one hand, I was fiercely determined to make a difference: *my* daughter was going to be loved and cherished in a way I never had been. Yet on the other hand, the realization that my mother had never wanted me hit me like a ton of bricks. How could anyone hate a cuddly little baby as much as my mother hated me? I was depressed for over a year."

Depression can be tricky to distinguish from other conditions that promote postpartum weight gain. A lazy thyroid or a post-trauma reaction can also masquerade as depression. But symptoms that should send you searching for answers include dramatic changes in eating patterns (either over- or under-eating); sleep-pattern changes beyond those caused by the baby (abnormal drowsiness or insomnia, for instance); frequent crying jags; anger attacks; an inability to bond with your baby; deep fatigue or lack of motivation; and intense feelings of worthlessness or inadequacy.

Since baby blues spring from so many complex causes, the solutions aren't always simple. But once you realize depression is at the root of your weight problems, you can start seeking help. Go to Chapter 10, "Losing Depression Fat," for ways to begin.

7. UNDERSTAND THE COMPLEX ROLE OF TRAUMA

The largest individual weight gain after pregnancy in one Australian study was by a woman who gained 150 pounds. Huge spurts like this often spring from some dark family secret, frequently childhood sexual abuse. During periods of great change and stress, such secrets often resurface, reigniting out-of-control feelings and triggering overeating as a way to numb the emotional pain.

One woman who'd been sexually molested by her father had no trouble with her weight after giving birth to two sons, but she gained more than 80 pounds when she gave birth to a daughter. (She herself had been a third child in a family with two older brothers.) Once she began working through the abuse in therapy, she was able to lose 60 pounds. Sexual abuse fat is, of course, quite complex. Go to Chapter 18, "Losing Post-Trauma Fat," for more information.

Surprisingly, a cesarean delivery, especially if it's unplanned, can also leave marks of trauma, making it harder to lose weight. For years, medical activists in the United States (which has the highest C-section rate in the world) have warned that doctors perform far too many of these surgeries without considering the emotional and physical impact on the mothers. In one survey of four suburban Detroit hospitals, 44 percent of first-time mothers over age 35 had C-sections. In Sweden, where these operations are far less common, researchers are beginning to connect C-sections with post-traumatic stress disorders. PTSDs typically spring from a sense of feeling powerless and invaded in a life-threatening situation. One month after their emergency C-sections, 76 percent of Swedish women had many PTSD symptoms, including unbidden flashbacks to the birth, anger, fears, and depression. Two months after surgery, these symptoms had often abated, but 33 percent of women were still suffering. In another Swedish survey, 55 percent of C-section mothers reported fearing for their own lives or those of their babies, 25 percent blamed themselves to some extent for the surgery, and 8 percent were angry, protesting they'd been very badly treated by the hospital staff.

How could a distressful birth make it harder to lose Post-Pregnancy Fat months after delivery? When you suffer a trauma, your emotional circuits become overloaded. Your cortisol highway, which starts in your brain, becomes "sensitized" and hair-trigger, reacting with lightning-quick speed to all sorts of stress. Even minor events to which you once wouldn't have given a second thought may now disturb you deeply. Such "threats" vary from one woman to the next. They can be obvious or quite subtle. You may find yourself dwelling on a negative newspaper headline, for example, or feel more deeply troubled than usual by a grisly story on the nightly news. Anything that reminds you of the birth experience—a baby's face in a magazine ad, the glimpse of a baby carriage, the antiseptic smells in a doctor's office—may bring memories flooding back.

Sometimes the memories themselves may remain buried, leaving you feeling agitated and out of control without knowing why. This uneasy sense of being hijacked by your emotions, in turn, eats away at your confidence. As Bandura observes, when we're emotionally aroused and have no idea why, our confidence plummets.

Joline, whose baby almost died during a particularly traumatic delivery, says: "For months afterward, I was hypervigilant, watching for danger around every corner. Just a car cutting me off on the freeway left me shaken and enraged. Any time I thought about the birth, I felt frightened, angry, or guilty. To soothe my agitation, I'd eat, usually some creamy, fattening food like ice cream or cheese." As you now know, extra dietary fat + cortisol = extra visceral fat. With the distress or low-confidence hormone often flooding her system, Joline's body might have stored more visceral fat if she hadn't consumed those extra calories. But cortisol *plus* ice cream and cheese was a surefire prescription for trouble. Eight months after the birth, she weighed 285 pounds.

Certainly not every woman who's had a C-section winds up traumatized and struggling this much with her weight. So if you feel fine, don't go searching for problems. Still, if you now realize you *have* suffered a birthing trauma, seek support, preferably from understanding friends and family. Take action. Just recognizing why you're upset and talking about your sense of being violated and vulnerable can help you work through your feelings. Remind yourself you *can* cope. Invent your own solutions. Keep an anger journal. If you're planning another child, switch doctors. When shopping for a new ob-gyn, ask about C-section rates. (A doctor with a high-risk practice should have a rate no higher than 17 percent; one with a low-risk practice, under 10 percent.) Donate money to a patient advocacy group working to prevent unnecessary cesareans. Do whatever it takes to assuage your feelings and get back in charge. Once you've reestablished your sense of control, you should find it a lot easier to slim down.

CHAPTER 17

Losing
Medication-Caused Fat

Drugs themselves, per se, have toxic side effects.
—*Neurophysiologist Bruce Pomerantz, M.D., Ph.D.,*
University of Toronto

Millions of women struggling with their weight have no idea their doctors are making them fat by prescribing drugs that promote weight gain. Of all the ways to be fat, this is undoubtedly one of the most common—and most overlooked. During the past year, just in my own personal life, I have met literally dozens of women struggling with Medication-Caused Fat. One mother was put on Paxil (a popular antidepressant) because she became justifiably miserable when her teenage son became verbally and physically abusive, and her timid husband did nothing to stop the violence. A second developed a round "moon face" and a fat tummy when she was given prednisone for an eye infection. A third gained over 100 pounds after having a hysterectomy (see "Another Way Your Doctor Can Make You Fat" on page 194) and going on estrogen drugs. To lose weight, each of these women dutifully followed her doctor's orders and went on a diet that didn't work. Yet *not one* of them thought about going off her medication. When we go in for our checkups, nurses waggle their fingers at us and tut-tut as we step on the scale at the same time the doctor scribbles another fat-promoting prescription! It's like a giant blind spot in our culture we need to correct.

Among the worst offenders are the tricyclic antidepressants, some of which cause weight gain in 89 percent of patients. More than 50 million prescriptions are written for these drugs in North America alone. Some women gain only one or two pounds on these drugs. But in one month, 28 percent of patients taking the tricyclic antidepressant amitriptyline (sold under the brand names Elavil and Endep) gained over ten pounds, no matter what their weight had previously been. When Madelyn H. Fernstrom at the University of Pittsburgh School of Medicine studied patients taking these drugs, she found that on some drugs, women's metabolisms dropped and on others their cravings for sweets rose.

Breast cancer patients frequently gain weight due to their medications. So do women with Polycystic Ovary Syndrome, for whom even the wrong birth-control pills can cause problems. Other weight-control saboteurs in your medicine cabinet to watch out for include prednisone (a cortisol drug five times more potent than the body's own cortisol); antihistamines (especially newer ones like astemizole or loratadine); anti-estrogen drugs like danazol and Lupron; blood pressure medications (particularly the beta-blockers); and many others (see "Fat-Promoting Medications" on page 199.)

How can you tell if a medication is making you fat? First ponder when you began gaining weight. Was it shortly after you started taking a certain pill? Most medications have so many side effects, it would take your doctor an hour to review them all. If you ask, "Will this pill make me fat?" your doctor may say no, simply because no patient has ever complained about it.

Now that you know how your fat cells work, you can also understand more clearly *why* a certain medication might make you fat. As we discussed in Chapter 6, the little fat cell doors called beta doors are the ones your effort hormones open to release fat. So when you take a beta-*blocker* for high blood pressure, guess what? The doors on your fat cells no longer release fat as well. Result: you may gain weight, even if you continue to exercise and eat as you always did. Cortisol, of course, also makes you fat—and so do cortisol drugs.

Another Way Your Doctor Can Make You Fat

It's common knowledge among obesity researchers that when a female rat has her ovaries removed, she becomes severely obese in no time.

After I recently met an extremely heavy woman at a health club who swore she'd rapidly gained 150 pounds after having a hysterectomy and even carried a pre-surgery photo of herself in her wallet to prove it, I decided to see if this phenomenon had been documented in women.

The evidence was buried, but it was there. In one international study by scientists in Australia, British Columbia, and the United States, women who had their ovaries removed gained an average of 11 pounds, although some individuals gained more. Surprisingly, those on the popular hormone replacement drug Premarin gained the most. In the Maine Women's Health Study, 23 percent of pre-menopausal women who had hysterectomies developed new problems with weight gain during the following year. Although some women mysteriously lose weight after this surgery, Nora Coffey, director of the HERS Foundation in Bala Cynwyd, Pennsylvania, estimates that the average weight gain after a hysterectomy is about 25 pounds. An estimated 20 to 25 percent of hysterectomized women appear to gain weight, mostly unhealthy apple fat stored in their visceral cells.

Why would losing your ovaries make you fat? For one thing, your metabolism drops on average about 100 calories a day when you're no longer ovulating. Though the effect has yet to be documented in humans, ovary removal in rats also alters levels of leptin, a protein involved in appetite and weight control. If you have only your uterus removed, will you avoid this side effect? It's hard to say. Each woman differs. In one Finnish study published in *Obstetrics & Gynecology*, however, women who'd had hysterectomies with at least one ovary preserved were still a lot heavier fifteen years later than women who hadn't had this surgery.

The key to preventing this problem is to become educated about all your options. A study in a recent British medical journal found that women with the least schooling were fifteen times more likely to have hysterectomies than those with a good education. In North America, high school dropouts also have this surgery far more often than college grads. As always, the best way to stay well is to stay well informed.

What You Can Do

As with other iatrogenic (doctor-caused) fat, your best choice is prevention. Once you stop taking a fattening medication, you can still lose weight. As Fernstrom says, "The fat's not cemented into your cells." But since weight loss is so tough, your best bet is to avoid, or stop taking, drugs *before* they cause serious problems. Here's how:

1. SKIP DRUGS YOU DON'T NEED

Doctors may believe they prescribe drugs based on scientific data, but many get their information from drug ads and sales forces. When UCLA researchers surveyed 109 drug ads in ten leading medical journals, 92 percent of the ads violated FDA guidelines: 40 percent of the ads downplayed the drugs' hazards, 30 percent cited statistics from less-than-convincing studies, and 30 percent included misleading tables and graphs. Drug companies also give doctors many free gifts including speaking fees, hefty "research" fees for little research, and travel to exotic vacation spots. One study showed that doctors who went on all-expense-paid trips to ritzy resorts, including a luxurious Caribbean isle, increased their prescriptions of the sponsoring companies' drugs by more than 300 percent.

Before taking any drug, ask questions: Has this drug been FDA-approved for your condition? Was it tested on women (not men) your age? How long did the tests last? Is the dosage right for your size and age? Will it interact with anything else you're taking? How will you know whether it's working? How soon can you stop taking it? What will happen if you *don't* take the drug? Be gently persistent. If you don't get a clear answer, rephrase the question and ask again. Also, phrase questions in a helpful, nonconfrontational way. You'll get a far better response if you say, "I have bad reactions to a lot of drugs—is there anything else I can try first?" Instead of, "Another *pill*? You've got to be kidding!"

2. CHECK THE PACKAGE INSERT

If you weren't given an insert, go to your pharmacist and ask for one (most pharmacists will be happy to give it to you). If for some reason you can't get a package insert, you can find the FDA-approved labeling for any drug in the *Physician's Desk Reference (PDR)* at your local library. Look on the labeling under the section "adverse reactions" (essentially, side effects). If weight gain has shown up in any controlled, double-blind studies, it will be mentioned somewhere in all that teeny-tiny print.

Don't be misled by how casually weight gain is listed. *Any* mention counts. Amitriptyline causes weight gain in nearly 90 percent of women who take it. Yet the package insert notes only "weight gain or loss," as if either one could happen to you equally often. Weight gain is also mentioned way down on the list under "other" reactions, almost as an afterthought, when it's a serious and pervasive side effect of this medication.

3. LOOK FOR SUBTLER HAZARDS

If a medication causes joint problems, depression, insomnia, fatigue, headaches, or some other effect that makes it hard to exercise or easy to overeat, you could gain weight even if the drug's not *directly* responsible. One potential side effect of the popular estrogen drug Premarin, for example, is "reduced carbohydrate tolerance." In plain English, this means your cells won't store carbs as well, and your insulin may become abnormally high, especially when you eat sugars and starches. If you read anything about the drug that disturbs you, call your doctor before taking it.

4. BE ALERT FOR DRUG INTERACTIONS

The more drugs you take, the greater your chances for "surprise" reactions, including possible weight gain. So keep a "health diary." Record any physical symptoms, mood swings, weight gain, or other side effects. Take the diary with you on doctor's visits so you won't forget anything you need to discuss. Also, recognize that you're only one of two hundred or so patients. Your doctor may not remember every detail of your care. When given a new prescription, mention any medication you're already taking; then ask your doctor if it's safe (and nonfattening) to take both.

Also, ask questions about any drugs prescribed for weight *loss*. The two drugs fenfluramine (subsequently withdrawn by the FDA) and phentermine were each approved separately, but the fen-phen combination was not. Prescribing drugs "off label" (for a use that's not FDA-approved) is perfectly legal but often unsafe. As we now know, fen-phen led to heart-valve problems in some women and even some deaths.

5. DON'T "MEDICATE" SIDE EFFECTS

Many people go on one drug that makes them dizzy, then their doctor prescribes a *second* drug for vertigo. Eric P. Cohen, M.D., of the Medical College of Wisconsin in Milwaukee, notes that a "plaguing symptom"—such as dizziness, fatigue, or high blood pressure—may not be some "new problem" that needs a second prescription, but a side effect of a drug you're already taking. He says, "What it often takes to clear up these symptoms is *less* medication, not *more*."

6. Don't Play Doctor

You may see one of your medications on the following pages in this chapter. *Do not stop taking this or any other drug without first consulting your doctor.* You may need to taper off slowly. Some drugs, such as certain antidepressants, can have severe *withdrawal* effects, including psychotic episodes, seizures, and suicidal tendencies.

Likewise, never pressure your doctor to give you a drug you've seen in an advertisement. Drug companies now spend over $600 million a year in the United States on direct-to-consumer ads for prescription drugs, thirteen times more than they spent in 1990. The drug may look good on TV or in a magazine ad. But a *Consumer Reports* survey found only 40 percent of direct-to-consumer print ads were honest about how well the drug worked and fairly described the risks and benefits in the main text. "I tell my patients the same thing I tell my medical students: don't get your information from somebody who's trying to sell you something," says Steffie Woolhandler, M.D., an associate professor of internal medicine at Harvard Medical School.

Also, be cautious about Internet promotions and "helpful" 1-800 numbers. The operators at the other end of the line may offer you "educational" pamphlets (put out by the drug company), medical studies (funded by the drug company), and physician referrals (to doctors ready to prescribe the drug with few questions asked).

Don't fall for it. Never press your doctor to give you a prescription for the latest "miracle" pills.

7. Ask about Switching

If you *need* a medication that's making you fat, ask your doctor if you can switch to a less fattening drug in the same family. Amitriptyline, for example, is a tricyclic antidepressant. So are nortriptyline, desipramine, and zimelidine. On the first three drugs, women gained weight (in a few cases, as much as 12 pounds in a month). On zimelidine, 69 percent of women had no change in weight, and 23 percent even lost a few pounds. Similarly, danazol, used to treat endometriosis, causes weight gain in more than 25 percent of women who take it, whereas Lupron (often used as an alternative) causes weight gain in about half that many.

In the end, you need a doctor who will work with you as a partner. Unfortunately, with so many HMOs now running the show in the United States, many doctors feel besieged. So you may need to assert your rights gently. Don't barrage a doctor who's running late with piles of medical-journal articles you've collected from the Internet. Also, don't assume you know all the answers (illness can be incredibly subtle). To avoid coming across as a troublemaker, prepare a list of intelligent questions and present them firmly but calmly. Ask your most pressing questions at the start of your exam (not as your doctor has one hand on the doorknob getting ready to leave). If any doctor treats you with disrespect simply because you're overweight, work hard to find a more compassionate doctor. You deserve it. A warm, caring partnership will provide your best chance for healing.

Fat-Promoting Medications

Many drugs can cause weight gain, but the ones listed below are some of the most common. Paradoxically, some of these drugs may cause one woman to gain weight, another to lose it. The questions to ask are these: When did you start taking the drug, and when did you start gaining weight? If the weight began slowly accumulating after several months on the drug, you may indeed have Medication-Caused Fat and need to probe further.

Antidepressants

    amitriptyline (Elavil, Endep)
    desipramine (Norpramin, Pertofrane)
    nortriptylene (Aventyl, Pamelor)
    paroxetine (Paxil)
    sertraline (Zoloft)

Anti-Estrogens

danazol (Danocrine)
leuprolide acetate (Lupron)

Antihistamines

astemizole (Hismanal)
chlorpheniramine (Alermine, Chlor-Trimeton)
diphenhydramine (Benadryl, Sominex Formula)
loratadine (Claritin tablets, syrup, etc.)

Blood Pressure Medications

beta-blockers like acebutolol (Sectral), atenolol (Tenormin), etc.
prazosin (Minipress)
terazosin (Hytrin)

Corticosteroids

betamethasone (Diprolene, Diprosone, Valisone, Selstoject)
dexamethasone (Decadon, Hexadrol, TobraDex, etc.)
methylprednisolone (Depopred, Medrol)
prednisone (Deltasone, Meticorten, Prednicen-M)

Diabetes Drugs

chloropropamide (Diabinese)
glyburide (Diabeta)

Female Hormone Drugs

conjugated estrogens (Premarin)
many others (check your brand)

Nonsteroidal Anti-Inflammatory Drugs (NSAIDs)

ibuprofen (Advil, Motrin, etc.)
naproxen (Naprosyn, Anaprox)

Other Psychiatric Drugs

chlorpromazine (Thorazine)
lithium (Eskalith, Lithobid, Lithonate)
perphenazine (Etrafon, Triavil, Trilafon, others that combine
  perphenazine with amitriptyline)

Sleeping Pills/Tranquilizers

chlordiazepoxide (Librium)
diazepam (Valium)
flurazepam (Dalmane)
temazepam (Restoril)
zolpidem (Ambien)

CHAPTER 18

Losing Post-Trauma Fat

One must finish with the past in order to go on with the future.

—*Therapist Claudia Black*

Caveat: *If you think—or know—you were sexually abused as a child but have not yet addressed the trauma, please do not read this chapter until you feel strong enough to handle the feelings that may emerge. It's best to have a strong support system in place or a competent therapist on your team. Suddenly uncovering a traumatic memory for the first time when you're alone and unsupported might release volcanic emotions that only make matters worse. On the other hand, if you know you were abused and are struggling with it, but you've never heard of Post-Trauma Fat before, this chapter is for you.*

Michelle, a New York City medical technician, is crossing a busy Manhattan intersection on her way to lunch. As she steps off the curb, a green Chevy runs a red light in front of her and zips on by. Michelle's not hurt. In fact, the car was at least six feet from her. But Michelle reacts in a very personal way. The green Chevy was exactly the same make and color of the car in which her uncle raped her when she was ten. Hyperventilating, raging, and shaken to her very foundations, she heads for the restaurant and orders the most fattening entrée on the menu, complete with a huge pecan bar topped with ice cream for dessert. She angrily consumes more than 3,000 calories before she can calm down. Michelle is struggling with Post-Trauma Fat, a legacy from a brutality she suffered more than twenty years ago.

If you, too, struggle with Post-Trauma Fat, you're not alone. Since the voices of the abused are so often silenced, you may think Post-Trauma Fat afflicts only a few "unlucky" people like you. Yet time and again, study after study reveals that 25 percent of women—and about 16 percent of men—were sexually abused as children. Nearly half of overweight women in one San Diego weight control clinic came from alcoholic or drug-abuse families.

Of all the ways to be fat, this is the most complex and disturbing. If anything in this chapter feels "not quite right" or a "little off the mark" to you as a unique individual, please disregard what's not useful. What counts are *your* feelings, *your* perceptions, *your* understandings. The very nature of trauma is that it leaves you with a system that's "on permanent alert, as if the danger might return at any moment." A large part of the process of recovery involves regaining your sense of autonomy. You need no "rescuers" to tell you how your life should be run or, for that matter, to tell you how to get thin. You need your own self-direction. When you have unhealed trauma, superconfidence when you finally achieve it is very hard-won, a true triumph.

Is This Your Problem?

1. Have you ever been sexually or physically assaulted (date-raped, molested, slapped, thrown downstairs, beaten with fists, or threatened with a weapon)?
2. Have you witnessed brutality, such as the murder or rape of a loved one?
3. Have you been in a natural catastrophe, such as an earthquake, fire, flood, or tornado, or been subject to a man-made disaster, such as a chemical spill or explosion?
4. Have you ever been in a war, a war zone, or a concentration camp? Were you ever tortured?
5. Were you sadistically disciplined as a child (forced to eat insects or worms, injure a pet or sibling, watch brutal violence)? Were you ever locked in a cage or a closet, tied up, or burned?
6. Have you ever been involved in a situation (such as a plane wreck, car accident, mugging, robbery, or emergency surgery)

during which you felt your life or a loved one's life was threatened?

7. Did you begin gaining weight *after* any of these traumas?
8. Do you suffer flashbacks or nightmares reliving these events?
9. Do you sometimes "numb out," suffer amnesia, or have out-of-body experiences, as if your body belonged to somebody else?
10. In addition to your weight, do you also struggle with other "inexplicable" symptoms (headaches, pelvic pain, heavy bleeding, mood swings, sleep problems, anger attacks, deep depression and despair)?

If you answered yes to any of the first six questions and also to question 7, you probably have Post-Trauma Fat. Answering yes to questions 8 through 10 means you have a full-blown case of post-traumatic stress disorder (PTSD). If you answered no to questions 8 through 10, your weight could still be the result of trauma; among sexually abused women treated for eating disorders in one European clinic, overweight women had the *fewest* PTSD symptoms, suggesting extra weight may somehow help you deal with the chronic hyperarousal and other bodily states that normally occur after a traumatic experience.

Whether you were raped; witnessed a savage murder; were sexually, verbally, or physically abused as a child; or suffered some other trauma, chances are you want nothing more than to put it out of your mind. Friends and relatives will probably agree this is exactly the right choice. They'll urge, "Just get on with your life. What's done is done. It all happened so long ago. What's wrong with you? Why can't you just forgive and forget?" You may even tell yourself that you have no problems, that "everything's fine."

Deep inside, though, you know that everything's *not* fine. You want to erase the whole memory. You long with a deep, wordless desperation to forget. And yet, no matter how hard you try, that's the one thing you *cannot* do. You keep telling yourself you're "just about to get it whipped," that any day now things will get back to "normal." Unfortunately, the combined experience of winners shows that to fully recover you must deal fully with the betrayal you felt, the lost trust you endured. You can't "just get on with your life" and blithely "forgive." That's not your weakness or "flaw." That's the nature of trauma. Processed in an area of the brain that has no words, traumatic abuse is truly an "unspeakable" secret. When society continually hushes it up (people don't *want* to know), it becomes even more deeply buried. This unprocessed trauma begins "eating away" at you in ways even you may not see. In a study at Brown University, 60 percent of sexually abused overweight women had trouble with bingeing, especially when they were anxious, depressed, irritable, or had just experienced a failure. Some women with Post-Trauma Fat are literally "eating their hearts out." The metaphor is real.

The Multiple Symptoms of PTSD

The three most common symptoms of a Post-Traumatic Stress Disorder (PTSD)—and also of Post-Trauma Fat—are chronic hyperarousal; psychic "numbness," during which you may drop into a trance (at which point you may eat); and unbidden flashbacks or nightmares. But each woman reacts in her own way. The long list of symptoms includes mood swings; body image disturbances; difficulties with trust, intimacy, and self-assertion; a view of yourself as "helpless, damaged, and ineffective"; anxiety; paranoia; and guilt. Perfectionism is also quite common. You may feel "I can't make a single mistake." Why? Possibly because when you let down your guard as a child, any misstep may have led to abuse.

Therapist Aphrodite Matsakis, who works at the Vietnam Veterans' Outreach Center in Silver Spring, Maryland, cites a number of perfectionistic ideas often accompanying PTSDs that put "an added weight on an already burdened psyche" (see how many apply to you):

I should be the epitome of generosity and unselfishness.
I should be the perfect lover, friend, parent, teacher, student, spouse.
I should be able to find a quick solution to every problem.

I should never feel hurt. I should always feel happy and serene.
I should be completely competent.
I should know, understand, and foresee everything.
I should never feel certain emotions (such as anger, jealousy, or fear).
I should never make mistakes.
I should have achievements that bring me status, wealth, and power.
I should always be busy; relaxing wastes my time and my life.
I should be able to protect my children from all pain.
I should not take time just for my own pleasure.

Although these "shoulds" are common to many women (not just those who've been traumatized), Matsakis suggests asking yourself questions like these: Were any of these ideas necessary for survival during your trauma? Are they still necessary now? Which ones would you like to keep or discard?

Aside from emotional problems and twisted thinking, other tragic aftermaths of unprocessed trauma include gastrointestinal pain (66.5 percent of women at one gastrointestinal clinic had been sexually or physically abused); insomnia, nightmares, and frequent awakenings (which may spark Night-Eating Syndrome); depression (which can lead to both Depression and Medication-Caused Fat); anger attacks (Anger Fat); and menstrual problems like heavy bleeding and chronic pelvic pain (which can ultimately lead to Post-Hysterectomy Fat). As you can see, nesting syndromes with this disorder are almost universal. Even if you don't remember the trauma (38 percent of women in one study didn't), "the body keeps the score."

When you're struggling with Post-Trauma Fat, you may be convinced you handle stress "poorly." But, in fact, for you stress is not just a *reaction*. It's a *condition*. Trauma often deregulates the cortisol highway and other body systems in a way that keeps your mind/body "hypervigilant," constantly on the lookout for danger. When you have Post-Trauma Fat, your mind/body easily shifts into a state of hyperarousal. When exposed to any situation reminiscent of the trauma (the glimpse of a green car if you were raped in a green car, for example), your emotional brain instantly shifts to a state of red alert, emotionally "hijacking" (as Daniel Goleman so aptly put it in *Emotional Intelligence*) the rest of your brain before it has a chance to think the situation through and respond calmly. You may also have trouble using your emotions as signals or as warnings to take action. Can you reeducate your brain or "rewire" it, if you will, so you *don't* have such hair-trigger responses? Yes. In fact, this appears to be what people who beat these disorders do.

Traumas can be overcome, or even prevented, so it's important to appreciate your resilience. Even in the most difficult of situations, the human mind has a choice. In Istanbul, Turkey, doctors carefully examined fifty-five Turkish activists (twenty-five of them women) who'd been captured and tortured, comparing them with fifty-five of their peers who hadn't been caught. These people had been exposed to extreme terror. They'd been beaten, raped, hung by the wrists, and electrically tortured. They'd had to eat feces in their food and sleep in vermin-infested surroundings. Overall, they'd been subjected to an average of 291 incidents of torture over an average time in prison of forty-seven months. Amazingly, only 33 percent of these tortured people had *ever* suffered a post-traumatic stress disorder, and currently only 18 percent had symptoms. More than 50 percent did *not* have nightmares, 76 percent weren't hypervigilant, 38 percent had no concentration problems, and 67 percent did nothing in particular to avoid remembering the trauma. Of the twenty-five women, only nine had ever suffered full-blown PTSDs, and only four—just 16 percent —were still suffering from this diagnosis. Women, in fact, did slightly better at enduring the trauma than men.

That's not to diminish the odiousness of sexual abuse against women and children. These Turkish activists were adults, fiercely devoted to a cause. They had a prior knowledge that they *could* be tortured, and they'd prepared for this possibility. That's quite a different matter from a helpless child who's abused, or a woman who's suddenly surprised by a rapist as she walks across a parking lot. How early in life abuse occurs also matters; the earlier it happens, the harder it may be to integrate it into your personality and view of the world. The element of unpredictability and surprise can also heighten traumatic symptoms later. Still, this study does show that severe trauma *can* be overcome. Even after the most brutal tortures, healing can happen.

The Paths to Recovery

Surprisingly, once you begin dealing with your trauma, overeating may be one of the easier PTSD symptoms to beat. Before you start trying to lose weight, however, you should be aware that fat may be cushioning you in some way from your pain. If you regularly yo-yo, this may be why. Matthew Clark and colleagues at Brown University found weight loss in abused women can often trigger memories, flashbacks, or nightmares—especially as they return to a weight at which they were exploited or when they reach any weight at which they feel vulnerable and unprotected. Some women may also find it hard to stop overeating when they feel physically rundown, uncomfortable, or in pain (with a headache, for example). "Weight loss itself," Clark and his coworkers say, "could promote depressive symptoms, resulting in a drop of confidence and even more inability to stick with an eating and exercise plan." When losing weight, slow and easy is much better for you than the blitzkrieg approach. Keeping a journal or recalling your past experiences with yo-yoing to see *at what weights* your anxieties begin to mount can also be helpful.

No one's pretending this will be easy. Nor am I presuming to provide all your answers. When you achieve healing, the victory will be all yours. Still, recovery tends to follow certain patterns. Here are a number of thoughts and winners' strategies that should help start you on the path to recovery.

1. PINPOINT YOUR TRAUMA TRIGGERS

When struggling with Post-Trauma Fat, you may have to handle all the binge-trigger emotions (anger, depression, boredom, loneliness, etc.) that other women face. (See Chapter 13, "Losing Two Kinds of Binge-Eating Fat" for this.) But you also have *extra* triggers you need to address. Anything that reminds you of the trauma—people, places, objects, even emotional situations that make you feel helpless, vulnerable, or out of control—may trigger immense anxiety and a binge.

Although each individual woman has her own set of triggers, these are examples of the kinds of triggers winners frequently report, situations that can sideswipe you by surprise, leaving you feeling jittery and unsafe, with your confidence shaken:

- Riding in a car or being in confined places like an elevator
- Lying in bed alone in the dark in the middle of the night
- Seeing red dresses (one woman told Matsakis, "I was wearing a red dress when I was raped")
- Eating anything creamy, such as puddings or ice cream (a common anxiety trigger in women who were orally raped)

As you can see, these triggers aren't "typical" for ordinary overeating. But they're perfectly normal for anyone struggling with Post-Trauma Fat. They're part of your body's natural defense mechanisms. You're not going crazy. On some level, your body (your friend, not your enemy) is just trying to help you survive. Your body has learned through hard experience that the world is a *very dangerous place*. At the time it learned this lesson, your body was absolutely right. But the lesson no longer works. Now that the danger has passed, your mind can reeducate your body to see the world in a more hopeful, loving, and trusting way. Once you begin recognizing your own personal triggers, you'll begin to see more clearly why you suddenly lose control for what seems like some "inexplicable" reason.

While looking for triggers, look, too, for anniversary reactions. One woman came to dread her birthday because she always gorged herself on cake and ice cream to the point she felt so sick she wanted to throw up. It was only years later when she realized her uncle had raped her on her birthday (telling her it was his "birthday present" to her) that she understood why. Sometimes keeping a diary of your binges and noting *when* they occur can lead to a breakthrough of understanding.

Will Therapy Help?

Many women with Post-Trauma Fat find therapy immensely helpful. The challenge is to seek out a therapist who will empower you to take charge. The current medical model in which the physician acts as the all-knowing authority will *not* help and may even set back your recovery. "Others may offer advice, support, assistance, affection, and care, but not cure," writes Harvard's Judith Herman. For a total healing, the "fundamental principle of empowerment" must be observed.

Look for a therapist willing to practice what's called "transparent therapy," someone who specializes in PTSDs and who will help you explore exactly how the trauma has affected you and let you set your own treatment goals. You need no one "manipulating" you or trying to "fix" your problem. You need to know exactly what's going on, so you can fix your own problem. Just as cancer patients who survive tend to ask dozens of questions about treatments and then choose those they feel will work best for them, you need to evaluate all advice until you find the strategies that work best for you.

Recovery can take place only in the context of a relationship, however. Since the damage occurred in corrupted, *de*formed relationships with others, it must be *re*formed in loving connections that promote trust, intimacy, autonomy, and initiative. Protective "rescuers," however "benevolent and well-intentioned," may do more harm than good, Herman notes. Any ally (therapist, friend, or lover) must respect your strength, stand back, and empower you to become the author of your own life.

Finally, any therapy that focuses *exclusively* on your weight or your eating behavior is too narrow, and any positive results will very likely be "superficial, partial, and temporary." In one study of binge eaters, 71 percent of those at high risk for treatment failure reported a history of abuse. To achieve lasting results, it's important to deal with the whole PTSD, not just your weight problem.

2. LEARN TO BREAK TRANCES

"When I ate, I was sometimes intensely aware of every bite I took, yet other times I'd gorge myself without even thinking about it, as if my body wasn't really mine," one Post-Trauma Fat sufferer reports. Another says, "When I ate, I'd just 'numb out.' It felt so good. After I'd consumed this huge amount of food, I'd snap back to my senses and think, 'Oh, my God! What have I done?' Then I'd feel guilty and depressed." This phenomenon of trance eating is a common aftermath of trauma. It's surprisingly simple to solve. The secret is to generate a list of strategies that might bring you back into the moment. What do you think you could do at these times to "bring yourself back" to the present and feel more centered? Many women find it useful to write out a list and keep it with them. One winner held an ice cube in each hand to break out of a trance. Another found she could "snap herself back to reality," as she put it, by looking at the date on a newspaper or on her desk calendar. A third made a tape recording of her own soft, reassuring voice, with a message that started like this:

> *My name is Elena. I'm thirty-nine years old. I live in Madison, Wisconsin. I made this tape on September 25, the day I vowed to take charge of my binge eating. I want to find better ways to take care of myself when I'm anxious. I know that I'm a good person. I love myself. I need to be gentle and nurturing to myself. Right now, I can do many things to make myself feel better. I can listen to music, go out for a walk, play with my dog, sit in the sunshine, phone a friend, light a scented candle and enjoy the soothing smell, play my guitar, go fly my kite . . ."*

She slipped this tape into a Walkman she always kept handy for emergencies. Whenever she felt a binge coming on, she listened to the tape. Another winner put about five minutes of self-affirmations on a tape: "You are beautiful, you are talented, you are worthwhile, you've just had a tough day, nothing's really wrong, etc." Then she recorded her favorite meditation music to follow, so that after listening to her own comforting thoughts she'd have thirty minutes of gentle music to soothe her. Any self-generated solution has a chance to work. Just remember the two rules: When you find an idea that works, keep doing it. When an idea doesn't work, try something else. As one psychiatrist puts it, we must become "the subjects in our own quests for the truth."

3. Use Your Secret Strength

If you often drop into a trance and then binge while you're there, you're probably quite imaginative and creative. This ability to "dissociate," or float free from reality for a while, can be a weakness if it dominates your life. But when controlled, it becomes a strength in disguise. It probably protected you during the trauma, so you didn't feel the pain so intensely. It also means you're highly hypnotizable and will respond extremely well to a self-healing technique called self-hypnosis, or guided imagery.

To try it, simply lie down or sit in a comfortable chair and relax. Breathe deeply. Close your eyes. Picture the most beautiful, peaceful, relaxing—and safe—place you can imagine. It could be a wildflower meadow, a mountain scene, or a lovely little church deep in the woods. It could be a place you know or one you've made up. As you envision this scene, use all your senses. If it's an ocean beach, see and hear the waves spraying on the rocks and lapping on the shore, watch the squawking gulls overhead, feel the sand squishing between your bare toes, smell the briny seaweed, taste the salt in the air. Vividly imagine this safe place in all its details. Go there regularly. Once you have this safe place deeply etched in your imagination, go there whenever you get anxious, agitated, or upset. When you feel threatened or sense a binge coming on, close your eyes, relax, breathe deeply, and go to your safe place. Stay there until your agitation subsides.

Dealing with Body Blame

"My body betrayed me," one sexually abused woman told her therapist. "How could I have felt pleasure from such a vile, disgusting act? It sickens me and I cannot forgive it. I stuff it all day long to keep it quiet." If you were raped or molested and your body sexually responded (a normal biological reaction), you might want to explore how you turned the blame for the abuse toward your own body instead of toward the abuser. You may feel that your body is "not you," that it "will never be good enough," that it's the "wrong size," or that it's not "worth" being nurtured. Just recognizing such feelings as the common, natural aftermath of abuse may lead to new awareness—and healing.

---

4. CREATE A LITTLE RETREAT

We've been talking so far about ways to make yourself feel *internally* safe, so your emotions won't sideswipe you by surprise. But you also need to make yourself *externally* safe. This is why during their initial recovery, many women who beat Post-Trauma Fat report creating a little "retreat" for themselves, a hideaway from the world where they can recover. Margery, who was raped at age ten by her alcoholic father and then *married* an alcoholic, eventually healed herself and found peace. But before she could do it, she had to divorce her abusive, 300-pound husband. Then she had to clean up her house. "After Bob left, we'd had so much chaos in our marriage, my house was like a war zone," she recalls. "It was an absolute disaster, and I simply *could not* keep it clean, no matter how hard I tried." A total clutter bug, she finally hired a professional organizer to help her throw out all the trash.

With her house tidy at last, she began doing more loving things to create a beautiful life for herself. She filled her home with the aromas of freshly baked breads and began listening almost continuously to music. Each week, she refilled a bedside vase with fresh flowers. She also lit scented candles in the bathroom, bought a huge fluffy bathrobe, and added a soft, cushy, floral comforter to her bed. Instead of watching the horrors on the nightly news, she read books by the Christian mystic Thomas Merton before falling gently asleep. In the winter, she learned to chop her own wood and built warm, crackling fires. "Bob had such a violent temper I used to be afraid all the time," Margery says. "Now everything about my little hideaway here makes me feel safe, warm, and secure." This was her first step in recovery, not her last. She still had much work to do in her retreat, as she began noticing, and working to overcome, her binge triggers. She also had to mourn the loss of her childhood innocence, her marriage, and the years she'd missed working to develop her art talent. (After all these years, she's at last begun painting again.) Eventually she has become strong enough to move on with her life in a gentler, more beautiful way than she's ever known. It's been a long, courageous journey. But she reports, "I've found out who I am, who I would have been if I'd never been raped." Also, as a side effect, she's lost 52 pounds.

5. REMEMBER AND MOURN

Harvard Medical School psychiatrist Judith Herman, director of training at the Victims of Violence Program at Cambridge Hospital and one of the world's foremost trauma experts, says, "Recovery unfolds in three stages." Creating internal and external safety for yourself (the process we've been describing so far) is only the first stage. The second stage involves remembering the trauma in all its details. The help of a supportive friend, loved one, or therapist as an ally during this stage is essential.

In her beautifully written book *Trauma and Recovery* (a godsend for therapists and women in recovery alike) Herman writes, "The descent into mourning is at once the most necessary and the most dreaded tasks of this stage of recovery. Patients often fear that the task is insurmountable, that once they allow themselves to start grieving, they will never stop." She cites the case of a seventy-four-year-old widow and Holocaust survivor who said: "Even if it takes me one year to mourn each loss, and even if I live to be 107 [and mourn all members of my family], what do I do about the rest of the six million?" Mourning is an act of courage. Even if you've remembered the trauma in painful detail for years, you may still have some mourning to do at this stage. Although recovery doesn't proceed in a linear step-by-step way, a good sign you've successfully traversed this stage is when you give up revenge fantasies and prepare for forgiveness. Forgiveness must not come lightly, however. This stage cannot be rushed. See number 4 in Chapter 12, "Losing Anger Fat," for more about the healing power of forgiveness.

6. RECONNECT WITH ORDINARY LIFE

In the third stage of recovery, both Herman and the winners report, you must develop a "new self." It's time to put the old life behind you and pour energy into taking care of your body, beautifying your life, making sure you're financially secure, and deepening relationships with those you love. One winner who beat Post-Trauma Fat says, "I was sick and tired of feeling agitated and angry. Then one day I thought, 'Okay, how would you *prefer* to feel?' I realized I longed to trust others. I longed to feel powerful and secure. Once I began focusing on those situations in which I already felt centered, safe, and in charge, I was able to see where my life was already working. That empowered me to make it work even better."

Many women during this stage choose to face their fears. One winner who was raped took a self-defense course. Another who had always feared she wasn't self-sufficient enough hiked the John Muir Trail, a rugged 207-mile trail through the High Sierras.

This is a time when winners begin taking great pleasure in just being "ordinary," in not having to watch every little step they take, in being able to let their guard down. One terrible aspect of trauma is that it makes you feel so "special." Everything in your life has to be at a "high pitch," or you feel empty and alone. If you're not creating some intense drama—if you're not fighting with your spouse, pursued by bill collectors, fretting over losing your job, bingeing on chocolate, or struggling with some other self-created "crisis"—life feels too ordinary and dull.

The final stage of recovery involves rediscovering joy in the small, ordinary details of life. In this stage, women who've beaten Post-Trauma Fat report taking exquisite delight in simple pleasures: the smell of coffee perking in the morning, the colors in soap bubbles, the patter of the rain on the roof.

In the end, the recovery from Post-Trauma Fat is about far more than fat. In fact, losing weight may seem insignificant compared to the real work that you've done. As the ultimate sign of recovery, a winner reconnects with herself. One incest survivor who had reached this third and final stage of recovery and had chosen to confront her family with the abuse told Herman:

> I had said everything I wanted to say in the way I wanted to say it. I felt very complete about it and was very grateful for the lengthy planning, rehearsals, strategizing, etc. . . . Since then, I have felt free. . . . I feel like I have a future! I feel grounded, not like I'm manic or high. When I'm sad, I'm sad; when I'm angry, I'm angry. I feel realistic about the bad times and the difficulties I will face, but I know I have myself. . . . I always wanted this freedom and was always fighting to get it. Now it's no longer a battle—there's no one to fight—it's simply mine. The final stage of recovery can be summed up in four simple words: Now I have myself.

Where to Go from Here

Post-Trauma Fat invariably involves nesting syndromes (problems with daily hassles, depression, anger, bingeing, and perhaps night eating, Post-Pregnancy Fat, and fattening antidepressants). So flip through all the chapters to see which problems you want to address and which strategies seem most right for you.

PART FOUR

Your Weight,
Your Way

CHAPTER 19

Designing Your Superconfidence Diet

Successful weight-loss programs are almost always home-built and custom-made.

—Psychologists Susan Olson and Richard Colvin

As you now know, the old calories in, calories out, paradigm wasn't totally wrong. It was right, as far as it went. It just didn't go far enough. Once you know why you've gained unhealthy fat and have dealt with one or more underlying problems, slimming down may still require dieting, or at least *designing a nutritious diet.*

What's the difference? "Dieting" in the popular sense implies eating in some special, unusual way until you achieve your weight goals (at which point you *stop* eating that special way and gain back what you lost). *Designing a nutritious diet* means trying out different plans until you find a healthy way of eating that you can stick with for life. Winners always make the second choice.

Contrary to popular myth, real diets *do* work. But you need to find or create the right plan—the one that meets your individual needs and works best for you. The winners have given us many keys to weight control, but one of the most important is this: the measure of a diet that works isn't how fast you lose weight or how much weight you lose, but whether it allows you to *maintain* a healthy weight. Any diet that lasts for only a few months or a year isn't a real diet. It is a trick, a con job, an illusion like pulling a rabbit out of a hat in a magic show. You'll often hear women say, "Yes, that diet worked for me, but I gained the weight back." Wrong, double wrong. If the diet *had* worked, the weight *wouldn't* have returned.

Did you ever hear anybody say, "Yes, that polio vaccine worked great for me, but I got polio anyway?" If a medical remedy works, it *works*, plain and simple. If a diet lasted for only a few months or even a year or two, it didn't work for you. It just temporarily looked as if it *might* work.

Women have been taught so long to blame themselves that when a diet fails you may even be protesting, "Well, yes, the diet *did* work for me, but I couldn't stick with it." And why couldn't you stick with it? Because on some unspoken level, something about that particular eating plan was not right for you. Maybe it left you ravenously hungry. Maybe it made you exhausted and irritable, wrecked your concentration, or left you craving some "forbidden" food. Convinced the diet was inherently terrific and you were somehow mysteriously flawed, you may have just quit, never thinking to reexamine the diet.

Happily, this will never happen again. Now that you're far along the road to becoming a superconfident winner, you'll find yourself adapting or discarding any eating plan that works only halfway. You'll simply keep searching until you find one that works completely for you. Why is it so important to individualize your diet? Because we each have different genes and individual bodies. So we each have different dietary needs.

Do It Your Way

Only you can know your own mind/body and how you respond to different foods. So only you can design a diet that will both control your weight and suit your unique health needs. For years, we were told we should all be on a low-cholesterol diet to protect our hearts. This blanket prescription led many women to stop eating eggs entirely. Does this mean when designing your own diet, *you* should stop eating eggs? Maybe not. Studies in the United States have shown that 50 percent of the variations in our cholesterol levels are genetically determined. If you come from a low-cholesterol family, you may be able to eat eggs without harm. If you have a family history of high cholesterol, even a little extra fat may send your cholesterol soaring.

Other studies have shown that 30 to 60 percent of the variations in our blood pressure have a genetic connection. These genes, in turn, may influence how we respond to caffeine. Some men with family histories of hypertension experience possibly dangerous rises in cortisol and blood pressure when they're under heavy job stress and drink lots of caffeine. If you lack such a history, you may be able to drink coffee all day at your desk without hurting your heart or increasing your rate of visceral-fat storage.

Is it important to drink milk or at least include plenty of calcium and vitamin D in your diet to prevent osteoporosis? Of course. Still, an Australian study found that 75 percent of the variation in bone density is also genetically determined. So if you have low-bone-density genes, you should also get plenty of weight-bearing exercise and work extra-hard to stay optimistic. Why optimistic? Because depression (high-cortisol-ism) leeches calcium from the bones as surely as a sedentary lifestyle or too little milk.

Should you eliminate salt from your diet? That depends, too. Some people are "salt-sensitive" and develop high blood pressure when they eat too much salt. Other people can eat salt and suffer no metabolic problems. Black people are more likely to be salt-sensitive than Caucasians.

Even wheat can be a problem for some people, albeit not many. A few "gluten-sensitive" people (gluten is a gluelike substance in wheat) can become so sick from eating wheat products they can die. This sensitivity afflicts only about 1 in 3,000 people in most populations. Among people of Irish ancestry, the rate is 1 in 300. My dad lost 40 pounds and almost died of wheat intolerance before his doctor figured out what was wrong.

Is sugar a problem, as the *Sugar Busters!* diet designers claim? For most people, no. For some people, yes. Eskimos have traditionally eaten very high-fat diets, getting only a scant 4 percent of their calories from carbohydrates. Now that they've begun consuming a more westernized diet, 7 to 16 percent of Eskimos have been found to have trouble digesting sugar. Women with signs of the Deadly Quartet are also advised to avoid sugar, because too much of it can elevate their insulin levels. Insulin alone does not make you fat. But insulin *coupled with cortisol* promotes visceral-fat storage.

Perhaps more important than eliminating every grain of sugar is eliminating diet sodas and artificially sweetened cookies and cakes. Mysteriously, many winners report they could lose weight only after going cold-turkey on aspartame-sweetened sodas and other so-called "diet" foods. As I read the medical literature, I discovered why. Substituting a low-calorie sweetener for real sugar may actually make you crave and consume *more fat*! Researchers at the University of Leeds in the United Kingdom refer to this phenomenon as the "sugar/fat seesaw." The more sweets you eat, the less fat you want, and vice versa. In one study reported in the official journal of the British Dietetic Association, substituting artificial sweeteners for sugar led to an increase of 11 percent in total fat intake. In the Nurses' Health Study, the strongest risk factor for subsequent weight gain was high intake of artificial sweeteners. Fortunately, as the scientist of your own body, you can easily check out this idea to see if it's true for you. Simply observe your own responses to artificial sweeteners; see if they could be contributing to your weight problems.

Should you include a few glasses of wine in your diet? As you now know, alcohol slows down fat metabolism and also raises your cortisol levels, so it's wise to limit or eliminate it when you're trying to lose unhealthy fat. Still, alcohol can have different effects, depending on your genes. Chinese and Japanese people appear to metabolize alcohol faster than Europeans do. After consuming moderate amounts of beer in one study, 83 percent of Asians flushed (indicating the alcohol was being rapidly metabolized), compared to only 3 percent of Europeans. Also, the more exhausted you are (from sleep deprivation), the more just a little alcohol will affect you.

By now, you can see why it's so crucial to design your own diet. Nobody but you can become the scientist of your own body and pinpoint your individual needs. Only you can experiment with different eating plans until you hit on the one that works best for you.

The Six Basics

Is designing your own diet hard? No. On the contrary, it's quite simple. The illusory complexity of many pop diets is only a razzle-dazzle smokescreen to keep you from seeing how incredibly easy it is to invent your own eating plan. We've all seen food, and we all know how to use it. There's nothing high-tech about this.

One good way to begin is to follow a pattern winners consistently use: start with six basic tenets of healthy eating:

1. Include plenty of fruits, vegetables (including dark green leaves), nuts, and whole grains.
2. Stick with lean meats, including fish.
3. Get plenty of calcium in dark greens and low-fat dairy products.
4. Eat mostly "healthy" fats (olive, canola, and walnut oils, for example).
5. Go light on refined sugars and flours.
6. Drink plenty of water.

Once you know why you've gained unhealthy fat and have dealt with any underlying problems (from stress to PCOS), these six basics alone may be all you need to get your weight under control. If you want to explore further, you can also look at the two types of commercial weight-loss diets available.

Only two? That's right. Although liquid diets exist, no woman can drink diet shakes for the rest of her life. That leaves you with only two kinds of diets involving real food: high carb and high fat. Both have been around for about 150 years. For more than a century, no viable new weight-loss diet has been invented, no matter what pop diet gurus may claim.

Do You Crave Carbohydrates?

As we discussed in the chapter on Binge-Eating Fat, no food is biologically "addictive." So strictly speaking, most scientists believe you can't be addicted to food. Still, you may *crave* certain foods. So do you crave carbs? Maybe. Each of us is unique. But it's far more likely that what you really crave as a woman is sugars and fats, says Adam Drewnowski, a University of Michigan researcher who has done some very good studies on food cravings. As Columbia University's Timothy Walsh has pointed out, Häagen-Dazs vanilla ice cream is 57 percent fat and only 36 percent carb. Even 40 percent of the calories in devil's food cake come from fat. (Men, incidentally, tend to crave salty fats like those in potato chips and pizza.)

To figure out if you truly crave carbs, Drewnowski proposes, just ask yourself this: when you're dying for a treat, do you really crave an apple, a plain baked potato, or unbuttered popcorn? Isn't it really doughnuts, pies, cakes, and chocolate (all those yummy combinations of sugars and fats) that float your boat? If you were truly a carbohydrate craver, you'd be hungry for plain rice, or maybe even fruits and vegetables.

The Two Kinds of Weight-Loss Diets

With hundreds of weight-loss diets on the market nowadays, how can I possibly boil them all down to two? Because no matter how you slice them, there are only three food elements on this planet: carbohydrates (which include fruits, vegetables, sugars, and starches), proteins, and fats.

It's hard to manipulate the protein part of the triangle much. A diet that's 80 percent protein doesn't exist. Why not? Because, with a few exceptions, most high-protein foods (milk, meats, cheeses, etc.) also contain substantial amounts of fat. When you increase protein, you also tend to increase fat. When you lower protein, you lower fat.

What about vegetable protein like that found in beans? Yes, vegetables *do* contain some protein. But no vegetarian diet can be classified as "high protein." By its very definition, a diet rich in vegetables is high-carb.

So we're back to our original statement. There are only two basic weight-loss diets: high carb and high fat. Within these two categories, you can fiddle a lot with the figures (that's what all the pop diet designers do). You can invent a diet that's 10, 20, 30, or 40 percent fat, etc. Or you can invent one that's 40, 50, 60, or even 70 percent carb. But you're still manipulating only two food elements: carbs and fat. The protein content will tend to rise and fall automatically, depending on how much or how little fat you include.

Once you think about it this way, pigeonholing all the fad diets on the market becomes baby simple. When you get ready to design your own diet or adapt an existing one to your own needs, you simply need to think about two food elements: carbs and fat. How low will you go on fat? How low will you go on carbs? These are basically the only two questions you need to ask.

1. How Low Will You Go on Fat?

You'll often hear about the virtues of a low-fat diet. To protect your heart, the American Heart Association recommends a diet no more than 30 percent fat. Many diet gurus go even lower than that, claiming we should reduce our dietary fat to only 20 percent of our total calories. Cardiologist Dean Ornish has managed to reverse heart disease (reopen clogged blood vessels) by putting heart-attack patients on diets as low as 10 percent fat. Ornish's well-known vegetarian program, however, includes many elements *besides* cutting fat, including exercising, giving up cigarettes, learning to relax, and finding inner peace. So it's hard to know how much of his program's success can be traced directly to fat reduction.

Just as some people are "salt-sensitive" and develop high blood pressure in response to an overly salty diet, some people are "fat-sensitive" and develop extra weight in response to eating lots of fat. In one study reported in the *International Journal of Obesity*, Swedish researchers looked at lean and overweight women who ate equally high amounts of fat. Overweight women were seven times more likely to gain weight on a high-fat diet than lean women, and those with family histories of obesity were *fifteen* times more likely to get fat by eating fat. So can you personally get thin by cutting fat from your diet? If you're fat-sensitive, maybe so. Certainly, many winners have achieved normal weights by cutting fat from their diets.

How can you tell if you're fat-sensitive? Winners simply cut back on their fat intake for a month or two and see what happens. If they lose weight, they stick with it.

Some women find they *do* lose weight on a low-fat diet, but they also get so ravenously hungry they can't persevere. Any suggestions? "Add more fiber," one winner suggests. She finds a really chewy bran cereal for breakfast, though not especially tasty, cuts her appetite. Another notes: "When I get hungry for fat, I eat a really spicy meal filled with hot, hot chili peppers—the hotter the better. All that flavor satisfies me so much I no longer crave fat."

Are there any dangers to going *too low* on fat in an attempt to lose weight? If you've already had a heart attack and you're under a doctor's care, maybe not. If you're healthy, maybe so. If you have normal cholesterol, especially if you're postmenopausal (lots of "ifs" here), new evidence suggests eating too little fat may make your cholesterol *worse*. At the Lawrence Berkeley National Laboratory (LBNL) at the University of California, Berkeley, researchers have found that there are two kinds of bad LDL cholesterol: really lousy, small dense particles (called pattern B, more typically found in men) and not-so-lousy large particles (pattern A, more typical in premenopausal women). When healthy men ate a diet that was only 24 percent fat, their large pattern A particles changed to the smaller, more dangerous pattern B in about 40 percent of cases. Worse, when fat was cut to 10 percent of total calories, nearly two-thirds of pattern A men experienced this change.

Does this mean an extremely low-fat diet can raise some people's risk of heart disease? So far, nobody's sure. But at this point, it seems prudent if you're healthy (and also postmenopausal) not to go overboard.

Rather than straining to cut all fat from your diet, you might be wiser to focus on the *type* of fat you consume. The old idea that all dietary fat is deadly has been replaced with a new idea that some fats are good for you. Monounsaturated fats like olive, canola, avocado, and soybean oils appear to protect your heart and guard against some forms of cancer. Conversely, saturated animal fats and really bad *trans-fats* (the kind in most fried fast foods, baked goods like doughnuts and cookies, potato chips, and other fried, crispy stuff) appear to post the greatest heart hazards. A review recently published in the *New England Journal of Medicine* noted that saturated fats like butter raise LDL, but trans-fats deliver a double whammy, raising LDL and lowering good HDL.

That's why a so-called Mediterranean diet—rich in fruits, vegetables, whole grains, beans, nuts, and olive oil—may, in the long run, be best for your waistline and your health. In a French study reported in *Circulation: Journal of the American Heart Association*, previous heart-attack victims who ate a Mediterranean diet were 50 to 70 percent less likely to suffer a repeat heart attack than those on a "Western" diet laced with saturated fats like those in milk, red meat, and butter.

Early studies showed the more fat women ate, the fatter they got. But more recent research in Europe (by some of the same researchers) shows high-fat diets may promote obesity only in women with fat-promoting genes. Further research in Sweden found dietary fat caused weight gain only in *sedentary* women. Physically active women could eat fat and stay thin. So if you're not fat-sensitive, perhaps your best solution is to worry less about fat and start exercising more.

What If You Ate Nothing But Carbs?

As you now know, the human body can't turn carbohydrates into fat. It's physiologically impossible. So if you ate nothing but carbs, could you eat 4,000 calories a day and stay thin? Theoretically, the answer is yes. But from a practical viewpoint, it's a nonissue. Think about it a minute. When you eat even one smidgin of fat in the presence of carbs, the fat gets stored as fat. You couldn't cheat even a little bit, or you'd start to get fat.

So how exactly would you go about eating 4,000 calories of *nothing but carbs*? You could eat plain pasta without oil. You could eat sugar—straight. You could gobble fresh fruits and vegetables and whole grains for hours. Four thousand calories is something like 50 medium apples, 165 tomatoes, or 200 cups of cabbage. You'd be stuffed—and sick of food—long before you reached your 4,000-calorie quota.

Going to any extreme when eating is a really bad idea. If you have any serious thoughts about doing something unhealthy like this, go to Chapter 13, "Losing Binge-Eating Fat," for help with normalizing your eating.

2. HOW LOW WILL YOU GO ON CARBS?

In the second commercial weight-loss camp, we have those folks claiming fat isn't the problem: *carbohydrates* are. Are they right? For some people—those who already have metabolic signs of the Deadly Quartet—maybe yes. But it's confusing. So let's sort it out.

First, as you now know, carbohydrates won't make you fat because you can't store carbs in your fat cells. It's physiologically impossible. So, on the flip side of the coin, cutting carbs per se won't make you thin. The real secret of low-carb diets is that they invariably also cut calories. Let's face it, when you eat no sugar and no white flour, you've pretty much eliminated all white-flour pastas, doughnuts, cakes, muffins, pies, and cookies. You're left with fruits, vegetables, and lean meat, almost none of which can be stored as fat.

For some women, a healthy low-carb diet (cutting back on the sugars and starches, while limiting fat to about 30 to 35 percent of calories) will also improve health. Why? Because carbs and protein raise insulin levels; and high insulin levels, in turn, can increase your risk of heart disease, stroke, diabetes, and some cancers. Sugars and starches—especially those in "fat-free" baked goods and kiddie cereals—*can* and probably should be eliminated if you already have signs of the Deadly Quartet. If you got a full metabolic workup as described in Chapter 7, you already know if you have dangerous blood abnormalities. If you didn't get a full metabolic workup, you'll probably want to get one. As we discussed in Chapter 11, the Syndrome X Diet isn't accepted by all the experts as the way to go. But if carbs don't agree with you and you're interested in a commercial diet, it's a good one to try.

Basically, Stanford insulin researcher Gerald Reaven maintains that if you have signs of insulin resistance or the Deadly Quartet, you need to cut carbs and eat more fat to reduce your risk of serious illness. He recommends getting a whopping 40 percent of your calories from fat, although other doctors say 30 to 35 percent may be better. Reaven's studies have shown you can improve your metabolic profile (reducing factors in the Deadly Quartet) if you get most of your fat from soft margarines and "healthy" monosaturated fats like olive, walnut, and canola oils.

Reaven's endless lists of recipes in his book on Syndrome X look like they'd be a nightmare to follow. But basically, if you eat plenty of fresh fruits and vegetables, whole grains, lean meats, nuts, and oils, you'll be on the right track. Eliminating refined sugar, flours, white breads, and rice shouldn't be hard. As one weight-control winner put it: "Basically, I just don't eat anything white (except yogurt and milk)."

In many ways, a well-balanced low-carbohydrate diet differs very little from a well-rounded low-fat diet. Both contain fruits, vegetables, lean meats, and the other basics. About the only difference each day may be the equivalent of a few tablespoons of olive oil.

Troubleshooting Your Plan

What if you designed what you once thought was the perfect diet, but now you're tired of it and just want to quit? Does this mean you'll never be a superconfident winner? No. It only means you're being human. You've run into an ordinary glitch. It happens to winners all the time. Wanting to throw in the towel is simply a sign it's time to confront some need you previously overlooked and find an innovative way to satisfy it.

One San Diego winner had tried numerous single-magic-bullet diets without success. She especially hated diet shakes. Finally, she was honest enough with herself to realize no commercial diet had addressed her two main needs: she had a sweet tooth, and she needed foods she could *chew*. Now she satisfies her sweet tooth by eating fruit with every meal and her chewing needs with a crisp luncheon salad. Another winner was hooked on late-night snacking. She'd always been taught she absolutely "must" eat three meals a day. It was her family's golden rule. But even after a healthy dinner, she could never stop snacking at night. Her solution: she broke the rule and began skipping dinner. Now she "grazes" from 7 to 10 P.M. on herbal teas, European coffees, and apples.

Another winner's chief problem was that whenever he had a sandwich for lunch, he also craved potato or corn chips, which he couldn't stop eating. "I knew that pigging out on chips could become an excuse for me to overeat and blow my whole diet," he recalls, "so I had to find a way around it." Once he realized what he missed most about chips wasn't the oily taste but the salt and the crunch, he was able to find a solution. Now whenever he eats a sandwich, he also has low-fat corn chips or pretzels.

Many of us believe achieving a healthy weight means giving up all fattening foods. But most winners still eat doughnuts, pizza, and ice cream; they just do it in moderation. Mary Anne, thirty-two, a restaurant manager and self-described "chocoholic," slowly savors one chocolate truffle every night before bedtime. This little indulgence keeps her from feeling deprived (she swears she also sleeps better), and she's still lost six inches around her middle. Pepper, forty-eight, a musician in San Francisco who lost 76 pounds, uses a strategy that works for many winners: she allows herself one "cheat day" a week (in her case, Saturday), when she can eat whatever she pleases, be it cake, fudge, or ice cream. Still other winners reduce their hunger by relaxing.

Eileen, forty-six, a kindergarten teacher in Mobile, Alabama, who has gone from a size sixteen to a size ten, says, "I used to come home from school ravenous and eat half a package of cookies. Now, whenever I arrive home hungry, I lie down, light a vanilla-scented candle, listen to Gregorian chants, and meditate. After about twenty minutes, my hunger usually subsides. Then if I still want a snack, I have a banana."

Certainly the stress reduction of meditation alone probably helped reduce Eileen's hunger, but that scented candle may also have had some effect. In a remarkable and admittedly baffling experiment, neurologist Alan R. Hirsch at the Smell and Taste Research Foundation in Chicago found that women who simply inhaled soothing, "satisfying" smells (a sequence of peppermint, bananas, and green apples) reduced their appetites and lost an average of about 5 pounds a month. Some lost up to 18 pounds a month. Why? Nobody knows. But Hirsch believes odors somehow "soothe" the hypothalamus, the body's appetite center. For what it's worth, as you'll recall, this also happens to be the place in the brain where the cortisol highway begins.

Winners seldom count calories rigorously. They prefer more permanent eating changes. But I did find a few exceptions. Eric, a computer-graphics designer from Florida who lost six inches around his middle, told me, "While I was flattening my stomach, I only counted the calories in meats, breads, pastas, and other foods I thought would get me in trouble—and I kept those to about 900 a day. Beyond that, I filled up on vegetables and fruits." This turned out to be a scientist-of-his-own-body stroke of genius, since as we now know, the human body can't turn carbs into fat.

So, to reiterate the point made at the start of this chapter, yes, becoming a superconfident winner may indeed require that you diet—but not in the old-fashioned way that involves tricking the body into losing pounds you can't keep off. As one winner told me, going on a one-size-fits-all ersatz diet "is like putting a Band-Aid on a broken arm and telling everybody you've fixed it when you know in your heart you haven't. By denying yourself healthy, appropriate, real treatment in the meantime, you're only letting the problem get worse." No, you want no outmoded Band-Aid jobs. No more half solutions. By designing your own diet, you'll at last find what the superconfident winners have already achieved: nothing less than complete healing.

CHAPTER 20

Becoming an Exercise Winner

Practice easing your way along. Don't get het up or in a dither. Do your best; take it as it comes. You can handle anything if you think you can. Just keep your cool and your sense of humor.

—Smiley Blanton, M.D.

We all know that exercise is the single best thing we can do for our health. If exercise could be manufactured, bottled, and put in a pill as an elixir for a long, youthful life, just a few tablets would cost a small fortune. Although working out may be a tediously slow way to lose *weight*, it's a good way to lose unhealthy *visceral fat*. It lowers cortisol levels, lifts depression, reduces stress, relieves anger, boosts confidence, and may even "remodel" your visceral cells so they release their fat faster. What's more, when you exercise along with your diet, you tend to lose unhealthy visceral fat *first*. That's why just a 10- or 15-pound loss can often reverse the Civilization Syndrome and all those signs of the Deadly Quartet.

Since exercise is so good for our health, why can't we stick with it? Happily, this is one area in which *I'm* a winner. That's right, lazy me—a woman who literally did not work up a sweat between the ages of twenty and forty-two—has now been exercising regularly for over twelve years. I've even written a couple of articles about it and had my picture published in a national magazine in my bathing suit, no less.

How do I manage it? Great willpower? No. In fact, sticking with an exercise plan requires no willpower. Like losing weight, it's a craft—a lot like tying your shoes, but more sweaty. Even if you loathe exercise as much as I used to, here are ten surefire ways to stick with it—from how to begin a new activity to how to get back to it once you've supposedly "quit."

1. START SLOWLY

Popular myth has it that sticking with a routine requires gung ho enthusiasm. Nonsense. If you can merely walk around the block or pedal the bike for five minutes those first few days, count yourself a success. Your best plan: establish *consistency* first and work for *intensity* later. When I first started swimming at age forty-two, I could barely crawl one lap across the pool. But after three weeks, I could manage six. Two months later, I was doing eighteen. And at last count, my lap total was 37,440—not bad for an exercise shirker. Another woman took it even slower: able to do only two laps at first, she added just one lap a month until she reached half a mile.

Will Exercise Lower Your Cortisol Levels?

Yes, but probably only if you're enjoying yourself. That's why it's important to choose a workout you love or at least like. If you think you "should" exercise but hate every minute on that treadmill, the distress you feel may *raise* your cortisol levels. Overtrained athletes—so-called exercise-aholics—often have high cortisol levels, and some even approach burnout. Here's the secret: if you're out of shape, your body may resist exercise at first simply because you're unfit. So to that extent, exercise at first may be a hideous chore. Once you've gotten back in shape, though, if you still feel *more depressed* after exercising than you did when you started, that's a clue you need to look for an activity you'd enjoy more.

2. EXPECT TO FEEL BUSHED

Avid fitness buffs insist that exercising instantly makes you feel more alert, energetic, and optimistic. Don't believe it. After my first 7 A.M. swim sessions, it was all I could do to crawl back into bed.

Only after swimming six months and boosting my distance did I start to feel better. Suddenly, I was able to walk faster and work harder all day without feeling tired. Fortunately, a friend had warned me about this initial exercise hump. Otherwise, I would have given up, figuring I was just too old and out of shape for exercise to do me any good.

3. Do Your Own Thing

If there's one golden rule to help you keep moving, it's this: choose a workout that suits your personality. If you enjoy making friends, you're more likely to stick with a sociable activity like tennis or a water aerobics class than a solitary pursuit like cycling. If you're highly competitive, marathon running might float your boat more than working out at home on a treadmill. If you're terrified of getting hurt, you'll find walking more tolerable than martial-arts training.

To tailor your workout to you, learn from your history. If you failed at exercise in the past, what went wrong? Was the gym too far from your home? Did your workouts take too much time from your family? If you fear the latter may be a major exercise obstacle (as it frequently is for women), make staying active a family affair. Push your toddler ahead of you in a specially designed jogging stroller as you run; go in-line skating with older kids; or schedule a romantic bike ride through the park with your spouse. You may even want to rent a bicycle built for two.

4. Know How to Blitz Boredom

I've discovered one surefire way to keep exercise from boring me silly: during workouts, I simply do something else to keep myself entertained. I love to daydream, for example; so while floating on my back, I often make up stories in my head. Or when walking outdoors, I concentrate on the scenery. One deeply spiritual winner uses her walking hours to meditate and pray. Another woman—a classical music aficionado—has lost 22 pounds listening to Mozart as she runs. You can't *will* yourself to enjoy exercise; you must find a routine you genuinely like.

Charlotte, a forty-two-year-old mother of three in Minneapolis, gets up six days a week at 4:30 A.M. (yes, it's still dark!) to walk about four miles with her friend Norma. On Saturdays, they're often joined by four other women and walk for three hours. Two things keep them motivated even when the temperature becomes frigid: feeling healthy and making *money*. As they walk, they carry along a plastic bag and pick up discarded aluminum cans. They then sell the cans to a local recycler and donate the cash to their church or another charity. "We have tons of fun looking for cans, it gives us something to do, and our walk is over before we know it," says Charlotte, who sometimes has a whole garage full of crushed cans.

Another boredom blitzer: vary your routine. Bike three days and walk two, run slowly then more quickly, follow one lap on your back with three on your side. If you have a favorite route you follow, reverse the route; or challenge yourself to find a new route each week.

5. Pick a Specific Time Slot

Exercising whenever you "have the time" practically guarantees failure. To turn exercise into a habit, the winners say, you must set aside a *specific* time to do it.

Rona, an exercise winner from Phoenix, manages to stick with her noontime routine by refusing to let other tasks interfere. She says, "All my friends and family know I exercise from noon to 1 P.M. Mondays, Wednesdays, and Fridays—*without fail*. If a neighbor pops in as I'm about to leave, I just tell her to make herself comfortable, have a cup of coffee, and I'll be back in an hour." By keeping her schedule inflexible, she's turned exercise into an unbreakable habit—"just like brushing my teeth."

Still, if you hit a day when you simply can't find the time for a large block of exercise, little snippets *can* keep you going. Whenever she finds it absolutely impossible to go walking, Betty, a thirty-six-year-old writer from a small town in Connecticut, tries to squeeze in exercise wherever she can. She says, "I throw laundry in the washer and hit the treadmill until the washer stops, do leg lifts during my lunch hour . . . anytime I can spare five minutes to exercise, I do it."

6. Work for Inner Rewards

Exercise will make your body look better—eventually. Exercising just to get thin or to look sensational for that class reunion will only cause your motivation to flag once your goal is achieved. Dreams of a perfect body have a purpose: they can get you *started*. But to *keep* exercising, you need to look for and appreciate more hidden internal rewards.

One of the earliest unseen payoffs for me came the day I was in a college library, the elevator was stuck on the ground floor, and I reluctantly began walking up four long flights of stairs. As I rounded the second landing, I suddenly realized I wasn't gasping for breath as I had in the past. To my delight, I was almost running up the steps and didn't feel the least winded.

After working out a few weeks, do you feel more optimistic and energetic? Do you sleep and concentrate better? Are you suddenly getting more done in a day—or making better decisions? Though nearly 40 percent of couch potatoes believe exercise will give them less time to work, in fact active women actually work two hours a week *more*, on average, than inactive ones.

7. OUTSMART YOUR "WON'T" POWER

Some days you'll resist exercising so much you simply can't browbeat yourself into action. In short, your stubborn "won't" power has won, and you know you're in trouble.

To overcome your lethargy at such times, break down your routine into small, simple steps and then do one step at a time. When the alarm blares at 5:30 A.M. and plunging into an icy pool sounds like the worst form of torture, I tell myself, "You don't have to go swimming this morning, you just have to get up." Then, "Just brush your teeth . . . just get dressed . . . just go start the car . . . just drive *past* the pool . . . just sit in the pool parking lot and listen to the radio." You get my drift. At every step (and this is important) I give myself *full permission* to skip out. By refusing to think ahead to that ghastly moment when I might actually plunge in the water, I coax myself along one step at a time until I finally find myself sitting on the edge of the pool. At that point, I figure, "Oh, what the heck, I might as well swim." That first dive into the water feels like an electric shock. But once I've conquered three or four laps, I feel energized and euphoric. The rest of the day, I congratulate myself on my willpower and impress (or annoy) all my friends by telling them I swam at 6 A.M.

8. TRAP YOURSELF INTO ACTIVITY

Many winners devise tricks to help them stick with it. Over time, they build confidence in themselves. One woman refuses to shower at home, so she has to go to the gym every day before work. Another, who wouldn't be caught dead at the office without her eye makeup, keeps her eyeliner and mascara in her locker at the Y so she has to stop there on her way to work. Other tricks: exercise with a friend and exchange gym bags so you have to show up or your pal can't work out; put three dollars in a jar every time you don't exercise, then hand over the money to an exercise buddy who *has* been diligent; keep a large chart of your progress on a refrigerator door so your whole family will nag you if you slack off; reward yourself with a "treat" (such as a new outfit or a massage) after you've exercised faithfully for a month. Also, never stash your gear in a closet (out of sight, out of mind). Instead, keep your walking shoes by the front door, your tennis racket on the couch, the jump rope in the freezer wrapped around the ice cream—wherever you'll see it and be reminded to use it.

9. Have a Backup Plan

However noble your intentions, life has a way of wreaking havoc on the best-laid plans. Health clubs go broke. Bicycle chains break and tires deflate. Pools close for repairs. There's only one way to keep exercising when unforeseen crises erupt: you need to go to Plan B. And that means you have to *invent* a Plan B—not "when the time comes" but now.

What will you do if you sprain your ankle while jogging? Will you lift weights while you heal, or use that rowing machine in the company gym? What if an unexpected spring blizzard buries your favorite walking path under two feet of snow? Can you use a nearby mall until the weather clears or pop an aerobics tape in the VCR?

When I can't swim (perhaps because I've strained a shoulder muscle), my backup exercise is walking. Living in southern California, I can walk almost every day of the year. And if I want to drive a few extra miles, I can even walk on the beach or enjoy watching snowy egrets while strolling through a nearby bird sanctuary.

10. When You Lapse, Don't Collapse

Lapses aren't just possible: they're inevitable. Most successful exercisers miss at least one session a week. When you falter, forgive yourself. What do a few days or weeks matter when you're building a habit for life?

Over the past twelve years, I've "stopped" exercising more times than I can count. When I catch the flu, go on vacation, or face a tight deadline, I've been known to quit swimming for a week or even a few months. I know from experience that the longer I'm off, the harder it is to get back. So the minute the disruption ends, I calmly resume my routine. I may have to cut back a bit for a while, perhaps swimming twenty-four laps instead of thirty-six, but within a week or two I'm back in full swing. Even if you've stopped exercising for six months, you probably still haven't lost all the fitness you gained. Once you get busy again, you'll be amazed how fast you rebound.

In the end, sticking with exercise doesn't require that you think, feel, or look like a jock. It merely requires diligently working to master a few simple skills *anybody* can learn. So let's hear it for exercise haters everywhere. Now quit complaining, and I'll see you at the gym.

Afterword:
Toward Health and Healing

For a large part of the twentieth century, women were told that even a smidgin of body fat was ugly and obscene. When we didn't buy that message (because we knew better), we were told we'd *better* pay attention, because that same smidgin of fat could also lead to a host of killer diseases. You now know this, too, was a myth. Yet many of us bought into the fear.

Once taught to distrust our bodies not as fonts of health but as sources of vile disease, we were then told precisely how and what we needed to eat to rid ourselves of unsightly fat and safeguard our health. We followed the prescriptions—or perhaps we should call them preach-scriptions—as faithfully as we could (some were quite convoluted). Yet we just kept getting fatter. The more experts we listened to, the more books we read, the more diet foods we bought, the more pills we took, the more out of control of our eating we felt. Convinced we no longer knew what to put on a fork or which foods to place in our mouths, millions of competent, adult women were reduced on a broad cultural scale to the helpless, infantile belief we could no longer even feed ourselves without the most authoritative guidance. Mothers who had fed newborns until they grew to the size of football linemen were told—and somehow *convinced*—they knew nothing at all about food, that some logician with a string of credentials behind his name knew far more about our lives and our bodies than we did. And we bought it. It was one of the greatest marketing feats humankind has ever witnessed, right up there with the salesmanship about the "glories" of war.

How was a whole society of the strongest, brightest, healthiest, most educated and creative women the world has ever known reduced to such a helpless state that we literally believed we could not competently nourish our own bodies without "expert" help? The latest "new rule" hot out of the nutrition labs is "listen to your mother: eat your fruits and vegetables." I recently won a $1,000 prize for a magazine story proclaiming this hot news. Why aren't we laughing at this? The idea that we were disempowered by our culture doesn't begin to explain what's happening here. As Eleanor Roosevelt said, "No one can make me feel insecure without my consent." We silently gave our consent and turned against our own bodies. But why?

Stress? Maybe. But that's too simple. Stress always springs from a threat we fear we can't handle. So where's the threat? Does this massive abdication of personal power spring from the fact that at least 20 to 25 percent of women in our culture (maybe more, nobody knows) have been sexually abused or subjected to prolonged, repeated traumas and left with an "imprint of vulnerability"—and that, in Judith Herman's words, "trauma is contagious"? Do even women who have never been personally assaulted empathize with our sisters, mothers, best friends, and daughters to the point that they still feel violated, attacked, and out of control, as if their bodies aren't truly our own? Or is it that we've lost touch with our deepest selves to the point that the only "selves" we can identify and mold anymore are those surface images we use to impress the world? If we view "illness as metaphor," as Susan Sontag so aptly put it, and if even unhealthy fat is stored energy (which it most certainly is), what does the virtual army of overweight women and men in our society today really mean? Are we choking down our energy and giving up in distress, because we think we have no other choice? Or are we about to release a flood of self-discovered *effort without distress* that will transform the world? If all the fat in all the highly sensitive overweight people in our society were not merely "lost" (as many would like for it to be), but vitally transformed into effortful, self-propelled action, what would be the result? What would *you* do with all that extra energy you've been stuffing down?

Are women in our culture really "over" weight? Or are we at exactly the right weights for the tasks ahead, the tasks we've been wordlessly assigned and only we can achieve? It was, after all, the

Duchess of Windsor who sniffed, "You can never be too rich or too thin." It wasn't a single mom with three jobs.

We're told that the deeper questions raised by the women's movement have been all but abandoned, that most women now just want to be pretty, sexy, and thin. I don't buy it for a minute. When women keep searching for weight-loss answers, I believe we're secretly searching for something far deeper than superficial diet promoters understand. When we begin asking why we're so fat and delve beneath the surface, we find not simply "too many empty calories" on our plates, but layer upon layers of stress, depression, trauma, rage, despair, and strengths without names. "Why am I getting so fat?" or "Why am I *still* so fat?" we keep asking ourselves. The questions keep tormenting us, because on some level we know the answers will lead to a truth we've been yearning to find. We know when we answer the "fat question" once and for all, we will at last come face to face with a creative integrity we need to assert. It's a process of self-discovery that could transform far more than our personal lives, so we must all do our best. Our bodies remember the answers to the questions we've forgotten to ask. You have the power. Keep searching.

Notes

Chapter 1: The Weight-Loss Winners

concerns about weight" were number one Linda Brannon and Jess Feist, *Health Psychology*, 2d ed., (Belmont, Calif.: Wadsworth Publishing Co., 1992).   *two hundred thousand studies and articles* From a Medline search I did on Oct. 8, 1999; these figures may now be much higher.   *Major international conferences* George A. Bray, "Historical Framework for the Development of Ideas about Obesity," in Bray et al., *Handbook of Obesity* (New York: Marcel Dekker, 1998), 22.

Chapter 2: One Size Does Not Fit All

Dr. Hilde Bruch wrote Hilde Bruch, *The Importance of Overweight* (New York: Norton, 1957).   *In a 1976 Dahlem Workshop* Claude Bouchard and George A. Bray, *Regulation of Body Weight: Biological and Behavioral Mechanisms* (West Sussex, Eng.: Wiley, 1996).   *Obesity is not a single disorder* S. A. Jebb, "Aetiology of Obesity," *British Medical Bulletin* 53, no. 2 (1997): 264–85.   *the "heterogeneous nature of obesity"* D. S. Freedman, "The Importance of Body Fat Distribution in Early Life," *American Journal of Medicine and Science* 310, Suppl. 1, (Dec. 1995): S72–S76.   *A study led by Elsie R. Pamuk* Elsie R. Pamuk, David F. Williamson, et al., "Weight Loss and Mortality in a National Cohort of Adults, 1971–1987, *American Journal of Epidemiology* 136, no. 6 (1992): 686–97.   *33,760 Iowa women* A. R. Folsom, S. A. French, et al., "Weight Variability and Mortality: The Iowa Women's Health Study," *International Journal of Obesity* 20 (1996): 704–9.   *At least six other studies* Tamara B. Harris, Rachel Ballard-Barbasch, et al., "Overweight, Weight Loss, and Risk of Coronary Heart Disease in Older Women," *American Journal of Epidemiology* 137, no. 12 (1993): 1318–27; Stephen Sidney, Gary Friedman, and Abraham Siegelaub, "Thinness and Mortality," *American Journal of Public Health* 77, no. 3 (1987): 317–22; R. P. Troiana, E. A. Frongillo Jr., et al., "The Relationship between Body Weight and Mortality: A Quantitative Analysis of Combined Information from Existing Studies," *International Journal of Obesity* 20 (1995): 63–75; I-Min Lee and Ralph Paffenbarger, "Change in Body Weight and Longevity," *JAMA* 268, no. 15 (Oct. 21, 1992): 2045–49; Millicent Higgins, Ralph D'Agostino, et al., "Benefits and Adverse Effects of Weight Loss," *Annals of Internal Medicine* 119, no. 7 (Oct. 1, 1993): 758–63. Many other studies have shown similar results, one of the most recent being P. N. Singh and K. D. Linsted, "Body Mass and 26-Year Risk of Mortality from Specific Diseases among Women Who Never Smoked," *Epidemiology* 9, no. 3 (May 1998): 246–54.   *American Cancer Society/Centers for Disease Control study* David F. Williamson, Elsie Pamuk, et al., "Prospective Study of Intentional Weight Loss and Mortality in Never-Smoking Overweight U.S. White Women Aged 45–64 Years," *American Journal of Epidemiology* 141 (1995): 1128–41.   *losing 10 or 15 pounds of healthy fat . . . may even turn it into unhealthy fat* Lauren Lissner, Patricia M. Odell, et al., "Variability of Body Weight and Health Outcomes in the Framingham Population," *New England Journal of Medicine* 324 (June 27, 1991): 1839–44; for a good review of the literature on the effects of weight cycling on your health, see Kelly D. Brownell and Judith Rodin, "Medical, Metabolic, and Psychological Effects of Weight Cycling," *Archives of Internal Medicine* 154 (June 27, 1994): 1325–30.   *62.5 percent had slimmed down on their own* Stanley Schachter, "Recidivism and Self-Cure of Smoking and Obesity," *American Psychologist* 37, no. 4 (April 1982): 436–44.

Chapter 3: Find Out Why You're Overweight
"life stress" as a major culprit Janet D. Allan, "Explanatory Models of Overweight among African American, Euro-American, and Mexican American Women," *Western Journal of Nursing Research* 20, no. 1 (Feb. 1998), 45–66.   *Kummerspeck ... gains that could not be explained by calories alone* Hilde Bruch, *Eating Disorders* (New York: Basic Books, 1973), 125–26.   *shortly after her father died Marilu Henner's Total Health Makeover* (New York: ReganBooks, 1998).   *One especially telling study* C. I. Fogel, "Hard Time: The Stressful Nature of Incarceration for Women," *Issues in Mental Health Nursing* 14, no. 4 (Oct.–Dec., 1993): 367–77.   *Ridha Arem, M.D. The Thyroid Solution* (New York: Ballantine, 1999), 30.   *Healthy Women Study* Katri Raikkonen et al., "Anger, Hostility, and Visceral Adipose Tissue in Healthy Premenopausal Women," *Metabolism* 48, no. 9 (Sept. 1999), 1146–51.   *Redford Williams estimates* Personal interview. Redford Williams offers a review of the literature linking anger with illness in *Anger Kills* (New York: HarperCollins, 1993). Another good review is Aron Wolfe Siegman, "Cardiovascular Consequences of Expressing, Experiencing, and Repressing Anger," *Journal of Behavioral Medicine* (1993), 539–69.   *University of London survey* Chandra Patel, "Identifying Psychosocial and Other Risk Factors in Whitehall II Study," paper presented at the 2nd International Congress of Behavioral Medicine, Hanover, Germany, 1992; published in *Homeostasis in Health and Disease* 35, nos. 1 and 2 (April 1994): 71–83.   *About 30 percent of women who show up in weight-loss clinics* R. I. Spitzer et al., "Binge Eating Disorder: A Multisite Field Trial of the Diagnostic Criteria," *International Journal of Eating Disorders* 11 (1992): 191–203.   *10 to 15 percent of women who try commercial programs* Susan Z. Yanovski, "Binge Eating Disorder: Current Knowledge and Future Directions," *Obesity Research* 1 (1993): 306–24.   *Binge eaters often feel warmer* C. Wayne Callaway (with Catherine Whitney), *The Callaway Diet* (New York: Bantam, 1990).   *Other signs of this common syndrome* Christopher G. Fairburn, *Overcoming Binge Eating* (New York: Guilford, 1995) and Susan Z. Yanovski, "Obesity and Eating Disorders," in Bray et al., *Handbook of Obesity* (New York: Marcel Dekker, 1998), 115–28.   *binge eater is more likely ... weight fluctuations exceeding 20 pounds* Sharon Alger, Helen Seagle, and Eric Ravussin, "Food Intake and Energy Expenditure in Obese Female Bingers and Non-bingers," *International Journal of Obesity* 19 (1995): 11–16, referring to Spitzer et al., "Binge eating disorder," and to M. D. Marcus, R. R. Wing, and J. Hopkins, "Obese Binge Eaters: Affect, Cognitions, and Response to Behavioral Weight Control," *Journal of Consulting and Clinical Psychology* 3 (1988) 433–39.   *45 percent ... reported ... dieting preceded their first binge* E. B. Spurrell et al., "Age of Onset for Binge-Eating: Are There Different Pathways to Binge Eating?" *International Journal of Eating Disorders* 21, no. 1 (Jan. 1997): 55–65. In a later Yale study (*International Journal of Obesity and Related Metabolic Disorders*, April 2000), 65 percent of binge eaters said a diet preceded their first binge.   *Ubiquitous Polycystic Ovary* Stephen Franks, "The Ubiquitous Polycystic Ovary," *Journal of Endocrinology* 129 (1991): 317–19.   *most common endocrine disorder* Andrea Dunaif, "Hyperandrogenic Anovulation (PCOS): A Unique Disorder of Insulin Action Associated with an Increased Risk of Non-Insulin Dependent Diabetes Mellitus," *American Journal of Medicine* 98 (Jan. 16, 1995): 1A-33S–1A-39S.   *as many as 80 percent* Robert A. Wild, "Obesity, Lipids, Cardiovascular Risk, and Androgen Excess," *American Journal of Medicine* 98 (Jan. 16, 1995): 1A-27S–1A-32S.   *Many are also infertile* This is well documented. See, for example, Dunaif, "Hyperandrogenic Anovulation (PCOS)."   *Evelyn Talbott ... was "surprised"* American Heart Association Press Release, "Higher Level of CHD Risk Found with Polycystic Ovary Syndrome," July 13, 1995. The study referred to is Evelyn Talbott, David Guzick, et al., "Coronary Heart Disease Risk Factors in Women with Polycystic Ovary Syndrome," *Arteriosclerosis, Thrombosis, and Vascular Biology* 15 (July 1995): 821–26.   *First described ... by Albert Stunkard* Albert Stunkard et al., "The Night-Eating Syndrome: A Pattern of Food Intake among Certain Obese Patients," *American Journal of Medicine* 19 (1955), 78–86.   *up to 27 percent ... 64 percent* Ibid., and Colleen S. W. Rand et al., "The Night Eating Syndrome in the General Population and among Postoperative Obesity Surgery Patients," *International Journal of Eating Disorders* 22 (1997): 65–69.   *75 percent of female recovering alcoholics.* Colleen S. W. Rand et al., "Patterns

of Food and Alcohol Consumption in a Group of Bulimic Women," *Bulletin of the Society of Psychologists in Addictive Behaviors* (now *Psychology of Addictive Behaviors*) 5 (1986): 95–104.   *higher-than-normal cortisol . . . low levels of melatonin* Grethe Stoa Birketvedt et al., "Behavioral and Neuroendocrine Characteristics of the Night-Eating Syndrome," *JAMA* 282, no. 7 (Aug. 18, 1999): 657–63.   *factors that can play into how much weight you'll retain* For a good review, see Lorraine O. Walker, "Weight Gain After Childbirth: A Women's Health Concern?" *Annals of Behavioral Medicine* 17, no. 2 (1995): 132–41.   *black moms are twice as likely* J. D. Parker and B. Abrams, "Differences in Weight Retention between Black and White Mothers," *Obstetrics & Gynecology* 81 (1993): 768–74.   *45 percent of women who quit smoking* Stephan Rossner, "Weight Gain in Pregnancy," *Human Reproduction* 12, Suppl. 1 (1997): 110–15.   *weight gain . . . in 89 percent* Madelyn H. Fernstrom and David J. Kupfer, "Antidepressant-Induced Weight Gain: A Comparison Study of Four Medications," *Psychiatry Research* 26 (Oct. 10, 1988): 265–71.   *51 million prescriptions* Marc Kaufman, "Newer Antidepressants Not Better, Study Says; Federal Analysis Suggests Fewer Side Effects Drive Popularity of Prozac and Similar Drugs," *Washington Post*, April 6, 1999.   *one weight clinic in San Diego* Vincent Felitti, "Long-term Medical Consequences of Incest, Rape, and Molestation," *Southern Medical Journal* 84, no. 3 (Mar. 1991): 328–31.   *Texas A & M study* David H. Gleaves et al., "Scope and Significance of Posttraumatic Symptomatology among Women Hospitalized for an Eating Disorder," *International Journal of Eating Disorders* 24 (1998): 147–56.   *Past sexual abuse . . . associated* D. M. Moyer et al., "Childhood Sexual Abuse and Precursors of Binge Eating in an Adolescent Female Population," *International Journal of Eating Disorders* 21, no. 1 (Jan. 1997): 23–30.   *of Holocaust victims* Personal interview, Rachel Yehuda, neurochemist and director of the Traumatic Stress Studies Program at the Mount Sinai School of Medicine.

Chapter 4: Superconfidence and How to Get It
Pam Grout Pam Grout, *Jumpstart Your Metabolism*. (New York: Fireside, 1996, 1998.)   *"the wind is taken out of the sails of anxiety"* Viktor E. Frankl, *Man's Search for Meaning* (New York: Pocket Books, 1984), 147.   *"high perceived self-efficacy" . . . more able to achieve* For a thorough review of the self-efficacy literature, including citations for all the findings mentioned here, see Albert Bandura, *Self-Efficacy: The Exercise of Control* (New York: W. H. Freeman, 1997).   *one classic study* C. A. Chambliss and E. J. Murray, "Efficacy Attribution, Locus of Control, and Weight Loss," *Cognitive Therapy and Research* 3 (1979): 349–54.   *Albert J. Stunkard and his coworkers* L. W. Craighead, Albert J. Stunkard, and R. M. O'Brien, "Behavior Therapy and Pharmacotherapy for Obesity," *Archives of General Psychiatry* 38 (1981): 763–68.   *reduced their binge frequency . . . by 72 percent* Albert J. Stunkard et al., "Binge Eating Disorder and the Night-Eating Syndrome," *International Journal of Obesity* 20 (1996): 1–6.   *isn't a global strength* Bandura, *Self-Efficacy*, 11.   *"biology of hope"* Norman Cousins, *Head First: The Biology of Hope and the Healing Power of the Human Spirit* (New York: Penguin USA, 1990).   *"biology of belief"* Herbert Benson, *Timeless Healing: The Power and Biology of Belief* (New York: Scribner, 1996).   *"biology of intimacy"* Dean Ornish, *Love & Survival: The Scientific Basis for the Healing Power of Intimacy* (San Francisco: HarperCollins, 1998).   *"biology of self-confidence"* "Biological Effects of Perceived Efficacy," in Bandura, *Self-Efficacy*.   *exactly the same biology* This amazing but true statement will be throughly documented in Chapters 5 and 6.   *so terrified of spiders* Albert Bandura et al., "Catecholamine Secretion as a Function of Perceived Coping Self-Efficacy," *Journal of Consulting and Clinical Psychology* 53 (1985): 406–14. See also Bandura, *Self-Efficacy*, 259–79.   *Catecholamines are the only hormones in the human body that play any serious role in breaking down fat. But when they rise too high, they can also stop fat burning* This is a summation of the information presented in detail in Chapters 5 and 6.   *"essentially mirror"* See Bandura, *Self-Efficacy*, 265.   *Situations . . . can be managed without physiological stress* Bandura, *Self-Efficacy*, 266.   *provocative study at Kaiser Permanente* Susan Kayman et al., "Maintenance and Relapse after Weight Loss in Women: Behavioral Aspects," *American Journal of Clinical Nutrition* 52 (1990): 800–807.   *Thomas Edison* Charles Edison, "It's Plain Hard

Work That Does It," *Reader's Digest*, Dec. 1961.   *Albert Einstein* Ernst Straus, "Memoir," in *Einstein—A Centenary Volume*, A. P. French, ed. (Cambridge: Harvard University Press, 1979), 31.

Chapter 5: Body Fat and Disease

doctors on the cutting edge For detailed reviews of this new understanding, see Bray et al., *Handbook of Obesity*. (New York: Marcel Dekker, 1998).   *25 to 35 billion fat cells ... 125 billion fat cells* Kelly Brownell and Thomas A. Wadden, "Etiology and Treatment of Obesity: Understanding a Serious, Prevalent, and Refractory Disorder," *Journal of Consulting and Clinical Psychology* 60, no. 4 (1992): 505–17. The calculation is mine, based on 35 billion stamps approximately one inch long, stretching 24,900 miles around the earth at the equator.   *fat comes in two colors* For good discussions of brown and white fat, see "Development of White Adipose Tissue," "Adipose Tissue as a Storage Organ," and "Brown Adipose Tissue," all in Bray et al., *Handbook of Obesity*.   *French physician Jean Vague* Jean Vague, "The Degree of Masculine Differentiation of Obesities: A Factor Determining Predisposition to Diabetes, Atherosclerosis, Gout, and Uric Calculous Disease," *American Journal of Clinical Nutrition* 4, no. 1 (Jan.–Feb. 1956): 20–34.   *an extremely thorough review* Ahmed H. Kissebah and Glenn R. Krakower, "Regional Adiposity and Morbidity," *Physiological Reviews* 74, no. 4 (Oct. 1994): 761–811.   *new ways of thinking* See, for example, Per Bjorntorp, "Etiology of the Metabolic Syndrome," and Ahmed H. Kissebah et al., "Clinical Manifestations of the Metabolic Syndrome," both in Bray et al., *Handbook of Obesity*. See also David V. Schapira et al., "Upper-Body Fat Distribution and Endometrial Cancer Risk," *JAMA* 266, no. 13 (Oct. 2, 1991): 1808–11.   *the "Deadly Quartet"* This term was first coined by Norman M. Kaplan, professor of internal medicine at the University of Texas in Dallas, in his paper "The Deadly Quartet: Upper-Body Obesity, Glucose Intolerance, Hypertriglyceridemia and Hypertension," *Archives of Internal Medicine* 149 (1989): 1514–20. See also Bjorntorp in Bray et al., *Handbook of Obesity*.   *free fatty acids directly into the liver* Many researchers have suggested this, but one of the clearest discussions is in P. Marceau, "Liver Pathology and the Metabolic Syndrome X in Severe Obesity," *Journal of Clinical Endocrinology & Metabolism* 84, no. 5 (May 1999): 1513–17.   *It may be other, confounding factors* See, especially, J. C. Seidell and Claude Bouchard, "Visceral Fat in Relation to Health: Is It a Major Culprit or Simply an Innocent Bystander?" *International Journal of Obesity and Related Metabolic Disorders* (1997): 626–31, based on a presentation given at the meeting on "Good Fat, Bad Fat" held in London by the Association for the Study of Obesity in Nov. 1996.   *Redford B. Williams* Personal interview.   *Bjorntorp contacted all the men and women* Per Bjorntorp et al., "Hypothalamic Arousal, Insulin Resistance, and Type 2 Diabetes Mellitus," *Diabetic Medicine* 16 (1999): 373–83.   *A study at Yale University* Anne E. Moyer et al., "Stress-Induced Cortisol Response and Fat Distribution in Women," *Obesity Research* 2, no. 3 (May 1994): 255–62.   *committing suicide* F. P. Heald, "The Natural History of Obesity," in J. Bastiaans et al., eds., *Advances in Psychosomatic Medicine* vol. 7 (Basel, Switzerland: S. Karger, 1972), 102–15.   *have fewer post-traumatic stress symptoms* Johan Vanderlinden and Walter Vandereycken, *Trauma, Dissociation, and Impulse Dyscontrol in Eating Disorders* (New York: Brunner/Mazel, 1997), 10.   *a well-publicized editorial* Jerome P. Kassirer and Marcia Angell "Losing Weight—An Ill-Fated New Year's Resolution" (editorial) *New England Journal of Medicine* 338, no. 1 (Jan. 1, 1998): 52–54. Many studies and reviews have supported the idea that weight loss may not help all overweight people live longer and, in fact, may shorten some women's lives. Just a few of the best of these studies or reviews include Reubin Andres et al., "Long-Term Effects of Change in Body Weight on All-Cause Mortality," *Annals of Internal Medicine* 119, no. 7, part 2. (Oct. 1, 1993): 737–43; Aaron R. Folsom et al., "Weight Variability and Mortality: The Iowa Women's Health Study," *International Journal of Obesity* 20 (1996): 704–9; Ancel Keys, "Overweight, Obesity, Coronary Heart Disease, and Mortality," *Nutrition Reviews* 38, no. 9 (Sept. 1980): 297–307; Susan C. Wooley and Orland W. Wooley, "Should Obesity Be Treated at All?" in Stunkard and Stellar, eds., *Eating and Its Disorders* (New York: Raven Press, 1984) Tamara B. Harris et al., "Overweight, Weight Loss, and Risk of

Coronary Heart Disease in Older Women: The NHANES I Epidemiologic Follow-Up Study," *American Journal of Epidemiology* 137 (1993): 1318–27; David J. Pettitt et al., "Mortality as a Function of Obesity and Diabetes Mellitus," *American Journal of Epidemiology* 115, no. 3 (1982): 359–66; Elsie R. Pamuk, David F. Williamson, et al., "Weight Loss and Subsequent Death in a Cohort of U.S. Adults," *Annals of Internal Medicine* 119, no. 7, part 2 (Oct. 1, 1993): 744–48; and J. Fuller et al., "Is Obesity the Risk Factor?" paper presented at an International Congress on Obesity held in London, Oct. 8–11, 1974, published in A. Howard, ed., *Recent Advances in Obesity Research 1* (London: Newman Publishing, 1974), 29–32. **the Fat Thighs Study** Richard B. Terry et al., "Contributions of Regional Adipose Tissue Depots to Plasma Lipoprotein Concentrations in Overweight Men and Women: Possible Protective Effects of Thigh Fat," *Metabolism* 40, no. 7 (July 1991): 733–40. **women with ... widest hips ... had lower rates of diabetes** David S. Freedman and Alfred A. Rimm, "The Relation of Body Fat Distribution, as Assessed by Six Girth Measurements, to Diabetes Mellitus in Women," *American Journal of Public Health* 79, no. 6 (June 1989): 715–20. **a cosmetic issue** Per Bjorntorp, "Visceral Obesity: A 'Civilized Syndrome,'" *Obesity Research* 1 (May 1993): 206–22. **recent notion that all excess weight ... a "disease"** Gina Kolata, "Obesity Declared a Disease," *Science* 227 (Mar. 1985): 1019–20. At the time a consensus panel declared obesity a "disease," Kolata reported that "although the panel was definite in its statements, the data it relied on in drawing its conclusions were soft, to say the least. Studies contradict each other, particularly in the area of obesity and heart disease." One researcher admitted there was no definitive data and that the panel's conclusion was based more on a "feeling" for the data.

Chapter 6: How You Form Unhealthy Fat Patterns

it all has to do with hormones For one good overview, see, for example, Per Bjorntorp, "Hormonal Control of Regional Fat Distribution," *Human Reproduction* 12, Suppl. 1 (1997): 21–24. **now-classic study** G. A. Rose and R. T. Williams, "Metabolic Studies on Large and Small Eaters," *British Journal of Nutrition* 15 (1961): 1–9. **food diaries** I. Romieu, Walter Willett, Meir Stampfer, et al., "Energy Intake and Other Determinants of Relative Weight," *American Journal of Clinical Nutrition* 47 (1988): 406–12. **gone into restaurants** M. Coll, A. Meyer, and A. J. Stunkard, "Obesity and Food Choices in Public Places," *Archives of General Psychiatry* 36, no. 7 (July 1979): 795–97. **peered into ... refrigerators** K. Terry and S. Beck, "Eating Style and Food Storage Habits in the Home: Assessment of Obese and Nonobese Families," *Behavior Modification* 9, no. 2 (April 1985): 242–61. **results of more than half a century of research** Meena Shah and Robert W. Jeffrey, "Is Obesity Due to Overeating and Inactivity, or to a Defective Metabolic Rate? A Review," *Annals of Behavioral Medicine* 13, no. 2 (1991): 73–81. **"they were probably right"** Eliot Danforth Jr. and Ethan A. H. Sims, "Obesity and Efforts to Lose Weight" (editorial), *New England Journal of Medicine* 327, no. 27 (Dec. 31, 1992): 1947–48. See also L. V. Campbell, "A Change of Paradigm: Obesity Is Not Due to Either 'Excess' Energy Intake *or* 'Inadequate' Energy Expenditure," *International Journal of Obesity and Related Metabolic Disorders* (Nov. 1998): 1137. **team at Laval University** Claude Bouchard et al., "The Response to Long-Term Overfeeding in Identical Twins," *New England Journal of Medicine* 322, no. 21 (May 24, 1990): 1477–82. **"nonresponders"** Claude Bouchard, "Individual Differences in the Response to Regular Exercise," *International Journal of Obesity and Related Metabolic Disorders* (Oct. 1995): Suppl. 4, S5–8. **their resting metabolic rates fell by ... 28 percent** Rudolph L. Leibel and Jules Hirsch, "Diminished Energy Requirements in Reduced-Obese Patients" *Metabolism* 33, no. 2 (Feb. 1984): 164–70. **undereating can alter ... metabolic rate** C. Wayne Callaway, personal interview. **and he's right** See, for example, Arne Astrup, "Dietary Composition, Substrate Balances, and Body Fat in Subjects with a Predisposition to Obesity," *International Journal of Obesity* 17 (Dec. 1993): Suppl. 3, S32–S36. **ten slender young transsexuals** Jolanda M. H. Elbers, Henk Asscheman, Jacob C. Seidell, Jos A. J. Megens, and Louis J. G. Gooren, "Long-Term Testosterone Administration Increases Visceral Fat in Female to Male Transsexuals," *Journal of Clinical Endocrinology and Metabolism* 82 (1997):

2044–47.   *men were given estrogen drugs* M. Krotkiewski and Per Bjorntorp, "The Effects of Estrogen Treatment of Carcinoma of the Prostate on Regional Adipocyte Size," *Journal of Endocrinology Investigation* 1, no. 4 (Oct. 1978): 365–66. See also Bjorntorp, "The Fat Cell: A Clinical View," in G. A. Bray, ed., *Recent Advances in Obesity Research II* (London: Newman Publishing, 1977).   *hormones may redistribute our fat* Mauro Zamboni et al., "Body Fat Distribution in Pre- and Post-Menopausal Women: Metabolic and Anthropometric Variables and Their Inter-relationships," *International Journal of Obesity and Related Metabolic Disorders* 16, no. 7 (July 1992): 495–504.   *Identical twin brothers* Bouchard et al., "Response to Long-Term Overfeeding."   *visceral fat in black women and white women* J. M. Conway, Susan Yanovski, et al., "Visceral Adipose Tissue Differences in Black and White Women," *American Journal of Clinical Nutrition* 61, no. 4 (April 1995): 765–71.   *two stress systems* For a clear explanation of the two stress systems and much of the material that follows in this chapter, see Marianne Frankenhaeuser, "The Sympathetic-Adrenal and Pituitary-Adrenal Response to Challenge: Comparison between the Sexes," in T. M. Dembroski, T. H. Schmidt, and G. Blumchen, eds., *Biobehavioral Bases of Coronary Heart Disease* (Basel, Switzerland: Karger, 1983).   *catecholamines . . . the only hormones . . . that strongly affect the dissolving of fat* Peter Arner, "Catecholamine-Induced Lipolysis in Obesity," *International Journal of Obesity and Related Metabolic Disorders* 23 (Feb. 1999): Suppl. 1, 10–13.   *double-edged sword* Arner, "Catecholamine-Induced Lipolysis."   *diet-drug combination fen-phen* Shauna S. Roberts, "Diet Pills for the Long Haul (Evaluation of Effectiveness and Safety of Long-Term Diet Pills)," *Diabetes Forecast*, July 1, 1996, 24ff.   *Cortisol works with other chemicals* S. B. Pedersen et al., "Characterization of Regional and Gender Differences in Glucocorticoid Receptors and Lipoprotein Lipase Activity in Human Adipose Tissue," *Journal of Endocrinology and Metabolism* 78, no. 6 (June 1994): 1354–59; and J. N. Fain, "Hormonal Regulation of Lipid Mobilization from Adipose Tissue," in G. Litwack, ed., *Biochemical Actions of Hormones*, vol. 7 (New York: Academic, 1980), 119–24.   *Cortisol-containing prescription drugs* Geoffrey Redmond, M.D., *The Good News about Women's Hormones* (New York: Warner, 1995), 37.   *after smoking just one cigarette* Ovide F. Pomerleau and Cynthia S. Pomerleau, "Cortisol Response to a Psychological Stressor and/or Nicotine," *Pharmacology Biochemistry & Behavior* 36 (1990): 211–13.   *one study of nearly two thousand smokers* Elizabeth Barrett-Connor and Kay-Tee Khaw, "Cigarette Smoking and Central Obesity," *Annals of Internal Medicine* 111, no. 10 (Nov. 15, 1989): 783–87.   *alcoholic men . . . compared to . . . teetotalers* H. Kvist et al., "Distribution of Adipose Tissue and Muscle Mass in Alcoholic Men," *Metabolism* 42, no. 5 (May 1993): 569–73.   *an influential paper* Frankenhaeuser, "The Sympathetic-Adrenal and Pituitary Adrenal Response." All the material on effort without distress, effort with distress, and distress without effort comes from Frankenhaeuser's work. For studies that linked the powerless reaction (distress without effort) to high levels of visceral fat in humans, see "Distress and the Deadly Quartet" in Chapter 5. Strong self-efficacy—or superconfidence—is an *effort-without-distress* (fat dissolving without fat storage) response.

Chapter 7: Do You Have Healthy Fat?

University of Massachusetts survey Lois Biener and Alan Heaton, "Women Dieters of Normal Weight: Their Motives, Goals, and Risks," *American Journal of Public Health* 85, no. 5 (May 1995): 714–17.   *Figure your WHR* Information for this section came from interviews with C. Wayne Callaway, Reubin Andres at NIH, and other leading authorities.   *Claude Bouchard* "The Genetics of Obesity," in Bray et al., *Handbook of Obesity* (New York: Marcel Dekker, 1998), 157–90.   *Factor in your age* This section is based on interviews with Reubin Andres.   *Find out your numbers* This section is based on interviews with C. Wayne Callaway and others.   *Look at your family tree* This section is based on extensive interviews I did for the article I wrote titled "This 'Tree' Can Save Your Life" (*Reader's Digest*, March 1993).   *First National Health and Nutrition Examination Survey (NHANES)* Tamara B. Harris et al., "Overweight, Weight Loss, and Risk of Coronary Heart Disease in Older Women: The NHANES I Epidemiologic Follow-Up Study," *American Journal of Epidemiology* 137 (1993):

1318–27. Reubin Andres et al., "Long-Term Effects of Change in Body Weight on All-Cause Mortality," *Annals of Internal Medicine* 119, no. 7, part 2 (Oct. 1, 1993): 737–43. *the Iowa Women's Health Study* Aaron R. Folsom et al., "Weight Variability and Mortality: The Iowa Women's Health Study," *International Journal of Obesity* 20 (1996): 704–9. *influential review of thirteen studies by Ancel Keys* Ancel Keys, "Overweight, Obesity, Coronary Heart Disease, and Mortality," *Nutrition Reviews* 38, no. 9 (Sept. 1980): 297–307.

Chapter 8: Choosing to Take Charge
When people are cast in subordinate roles Bandura, *Self-Efficacy*, 18. *pseudo-incompetence sets in* Ibid. *seeing an overweight woman* B. L. Green and D. S. Saenz, "Tests of a Mediational Model of Restrained Eating: The Role of Dieting Self-Efficacy and Social Comparisons," *Journal of Social and Clinical Psychology* 14 (1995): 1–22. *Vincent J. Felliti* Personal interview. *"the second shift,"* Arlie Hochschild, *The Second Shift* (New York: Avon, 1997). *dinnertime conversations* Richard B. Stuart and Barbara Jacobson, *Weight, Sex, and Marriage: A Delicate Balance* (New York: Guilford, 1995). *another survey by Stuart* Ibid. *the "Little Red Hen" transition* Robert H. Colvin and Susan C. Olson, *Keeping It Off* (New York: Simon and Schuster, 1983), 29. *Mindfulness ... alter that same part of the brain* Joan Borysenko, *Minding the Body, Mending the Mind* (New York: Bantam, Doubleday, Dell, 1993).

Chapter 9: Losing Daily Hassles Fat
University of California at Berkeley study Anita DeLongis et al., "Relationship of Daily Hassles, Uplifts, and Major Life Events to Health Status," *Health Psychology* 1, no. 2 (1982): 119–36. *Matthew M. Clark at Brown University* Matthew M. Clark et al., "Self-Efficacy in Weight Management," *Journal of Consulting and Clinical Psychology* 39, no. 5 (1991): 739–44. *women who continued to lose weight* Deborah J. Kennett and Marilyn Ackerman, "Importance of Learned Resourcefulness to Weight Loss and Early Success during Maintenance: Preliminary Evidence," *Patient Education and Counseling* 25 (1995): 197–203. *fourteen minutes of negative news* Wendy M. Johnston and Graham C. L. Davey, "The Psychological Impact of Negative TV News Bulletins: The Catastrophizing of Personal Worries," *British Medical Journal* 88, Part 1 (Feb. 1997): 85–91. *one Italian study* G. Gerra et al., "Neuroendocrine Responses to Emotional Arousal in Normal Women," *Neuropsychobiology* 33, no. 4 (1996): 173–81. *women eat more fattening foods* Kelly Brownell and Elissa Epel, paper presented at the 19th annual meeting of the Society of Behavioral Medicine in March, 1998 in New Orleans. *a University of Kansas study* Sue Popkess-Vawter et al., "Overeating, Reversal Theory, and Weight Cycling," *Western Journal of Nursing Research* 20, no. 1 (1998): 67–83. *Cigarette smokers ... have more unhealthy visceral fat than nonsmokers* Elizabeth Barrett-Connor and Kay-Tee Khaw, "Cigarette Smoking and Central Obesity," *Annals of Internal Medicine* 111, no. 10 (Nov. 15, 1989): 783–87. *your body has no ... alcohol-storage compartments* Andrew M. Prentice, "Alcohol and Obesity," *International Journal of Obesity* 19 (1995): Suppl. 5, S44–S50. *Swiss study reported in the* New England Journal of Medicine Paolo M. Suter et al., "The Effect of Ethanol on Fat Storage in Healthy Subjects," 326, no. 15 (April 9, 1992): 983–87. *a study done at King's College* A. G. Dulloo et al., "Normal Caffeine Consumption: Influence on Thermogenesis and Daily Energy Expenditure in Lean and Postobese Human Volunteers," *American Journal of Clinical Nutrition* 49, no. 1 (Jan. 1989): 44–50. *a "caffeine-sensitive" subgroup* William R. Lovallo, "Caffeine May Potentiate Adrenocortical Stress Responses in Hypertension-Prone Men," *Hypertension* 14, no. 2 (Aug. 1989): 170–76.

Chapter 10: Losing Depression Fat
forty-nine out of seventy-six patients ... had been wait-listed H. E. R. Wallace and M. B. H. Whyte, "Natural History of the Psychoneuroses," *British Medical Journal* 1 (1959): 144. *an investigation by researchers at Duke University* J. C. Barefoot and M. Schroll, "Symptoms of Depression,

Acute Myocardial Infarction, and Total Mortality in a Community Sample," *Circulation* 93, no. 11 (June 1, 1996): 1976–80.   *Robert Thayer* personal interview.   *peak between 11 A.M. and 1 P.M. . . . lowest . . . 11 P.M.* Ibid.   *short but strenuous workouts* J. A. Blumenthal et al., "Effects of Exercise Training on Older Patients with Major Depression," *Archives of Internal Medicine* 159, no. 19 (Oct. 1999): 2349–56.   *optimism is learned in three ways* Martin E. P. Seligman, *Learned Optimism* (New York: Knopf, 1991).   *57 percent . . . eat sweets . . . 14 percent drink alcohol* Kurt Krauchi et al., "Eating Style in Seasonal Affective Disorder: Who Will Gain Weight in Winter?" *Comprehensive Psychiatry* 38, no. 2 (March/April 1997): 80–87.   *17 percent* Atezaz Saeed and Timothy J. Bruce, "Seasonal Affective Disorders," *American Family Physician* 57, no. 6 (Mar. 15, 1998): 1340–46, 1351–52.   *To find relief* These tips originally appeared in "Diet Traps," an article I wrote for *Woman's Day*, April 23, 1996.   *compared St. John's wort with Prozac* E. Schrader, "Equivalence of St. John's Wort Extract (Ze 117) and Fluoxetine: A Randomized, Controlled Study in Mild-Moderate Depression, *International Clinical Psychopharmacology* 15, no. 2 (Mar. 2000): 61–68.   *dose of St. John's wort* M. Philipp et al., "Hypericum Extract Versus Imipramine or Placebo in Patients with Moderate Depression; Randomized Multicentre Study of Treatment for Eight Weeks," *British Medical Journal* 319 (Dec. 11, 1999): 1534–38.   *"gaslighting"* George R. Bach and Peter Wyden, *The Intimate Enemy: How to Fight Fair in Love and Marriage* (New York: William Morrow, 1969).   *many categories of verbal abuse* Patricia Evans, *The Verbally Abusive Relationship: How to Recognize It and How to Respond* (Holbrook, Mass: Adams, 1992).

Chapter 11: Losing Lazy Thyroid Fat

one in ten . . . half . . . have no idea All the statistics in this paragraph come from the Feb. 28, 2000, issue of *Archives of Internal Medicine* and an *Archives of Internal Medicine/Medscape Wire*, "Study Shows Twice as Many Americans May Suffer from Undiagnosed Thyroid Disease," Mar. 2, 2000.   *your risk of heart disease rises* *Archives of Internal Medicine*, Feb. 28, 2000.   *simple, home self-test* This is a fairly common test, suggested in a number of places. See, for example, James F. Balch, M.D., and Phyllis A. Balch, *Prescription for Nutritional Healing* (Garden City Park, N.Y.: Avery, 1997).   *the usual treatment* For reliable information about hypothyroidism, start with the Thyroid Foundation of America at 800-832-8321, or visit their Web site at *http://www.tsh.org*. Information about thyroid disorders and physician referrals can also be obtained from the American Foundation of Thyroid Patients at 888-996-4460. Their Web site is thyroidfoundation.org.   *best to start low and work up* from Public Citizen's Sidney Wolfe, M.D., lead author of *Worst Pills, Best Pills*.   *avoid cheaper generics* Thyroid drugs must be very delicately matched to individual patients' needs; just a small variation can throw off the balance.

    American College of Physicians See Position Papers: "Screening for Thyroid Disease," *Annals of Internal Medicine* 129 (July 15, 1998): 141–43 and an accompanying article, 144–58.   *some patient activists* Personal interviews.   *Too much thyroid hormone* See Public Citizen's *Worst Pills, Best Pills*.   *women . . . treated with a T-4/T-3 combination* Robertas Bunevicius et al., "Effects of Thyroxine as Compared with Thyroxine plus Triiodothyronine in Patients with Hypothyroidism," *New England Journal of Medicine* 340, no. 6 (Feb. 11, 1999): 424–29.   *Syndrome X Diet* Reaven still believes "a calorie is a calorie is a calorie." He's not an obesity researcher. But when he talks about insulin and Syndrome X (the term he himself coined), he's worth listening to. You may want to pick up his book *Syndrome X* (New York: Simon & Schuster, 2000) at a library.   *Broda O. Barnes, M.D.* Broda O. Barnes, *Hypothyroidism: The Unsuspected Illness* (New York: Harper & Row, 1976). This book is interesting because it's so detailed and readable, but it *is* extremely outdated. So take anything you read here as a first step for asking questions, not as a final answer of any kind.   *East German refugees* M. Bauer et al., "Psychological and Endocrine Abnormalities in Refugees from East Germany: Part I. Prolonged Stress, Psychopathology, and Hypothalamic-Pituitary-Thyroid Axis Activity," *Psychiatry Research* 51, no. 1 (Jan. 1994): 61–73.

Chapter 12: Losing Anger Fat

talk show host Rosie O'Donnell Mary Duffy, "Role Models for Fitness Now Come in Super Sizes," *New York Times*, Dec. 28, 1999. *108 American women* Rena R. Wing et al., "Waist to Hip Ratio in Middle-Aged Women: Associations with Behavioral and Psychosocial Factors and with Changes in Cardiovascular Risk Factors," *Arteriosclerosis and Thrombosis* 11, no. 5 (Sept./Oct. 1991): 1250–57. *University of Utah study* Mary Katherine Pope and Timothy W. Smith, "Cortisol Excretion in High and Low Cynically Hostile Men," *Psychosomatic Medicine* 53 (1991): 386–92. *high blood pressure ... high insulin levels* Edward C. Suarez et al., "The Relation of Hostility to Lipids and Lipidproteins in Women: Evidence for the Role of Antagonistic Hostility," *Annals of Behavioral Medicine* 20, no. 2 (1998): 59–63; Katri Raikkonen et al., "The Role of Psychological Coronary Risk Factors in Insulin and Glucose Metabolism," *Journal of Psychosomatic Research* 38, no. 7 (Oct. 1993): 705–13; David Shapiro et al., "Effects of Cynical Hostility, Anger Out, Anxiety, and Defensiveness on Ambulatory Blood Pressure in Black and White College Students," *Psychosomatic Medicine* 58 (1996): 354–64; Liisa Keltikangas-Jarvinen et al., "Vital Exhaustion, Anger Expression, and Pituitary and Adrenocortical Hormones: Implications for the Insulin Resistance Syndrome," *Arteriosclerosis, Thrombosis, and Vascular Biology* 16, no. 2 (Feb. 1996): 275–80. Many other studies have linked heart-disease risk factors with anger. *600 more calories* Larry W. Scherwitz et al., "Hostility and Health Behaviors in Young Adults: The CARDIA Study," *American Journal of Epidemiology* 136 (1992): 136–45. *anger can redistribute your fat* Redford Williams, personal interview. *series of Harvard Medical School studies* Maurizio Fava et al., "Anger Attacks in Eating Disorders," *Psychiatry Research* 56 (1995): 205–12; Fava et al., "Anger Attacks in Depressed Outpatients," *Psychopharmacology Bulletin* 27 (1991): 275–79. *Redford Williams estimates* Personal interview. For more about the dangers of anger to your heart, see Williams's book *Anger Kills*, written with Virginia Williams (New York: HarperCollins, 1993). *multiple ways to be angry* Howard S. Friedman et al., "Personality Dimensions and Measures Potentially Relevant to Health: A Focus on Hostility," *Annals of Behavioral Medicine* 17, no. 3 (1995): 245–53. *hostile women consumed more animal fat ... men also ate more sugar* Linda Musante et al., "Hostility: Relationship to Lifestyle Behaviors and Physical Risk Factors," *Behavioral Medicine* 18 (Spring 1992): 21–26. *anger-out was the culprit* Katri Raikkonen et al., "Anger, Hostility, and Visceral Adipose Tissue in Healthy Postmenopausal Women," *Metabolism* 48, no. 9 (Sept. 1999): 1146–51. *Women's Anger Study* S. Thomas et al., "It Hurts Most around the Heart: A Phenomenological Exploration of Women's Anger," *Journal of Advanced Nursing* 28, no. 2 (Aug. 1998): 311–22. *"the right to be the final judge of yourself"* Manuel J. Smith, Ph.D., *When I Say No, I Feel Guilty* (New York: Bantam, 1975). *unhappily married ... gained ... 42½ pounds* Stuart and Jacobson (1987). *men pull the old "silent treatment" routine* John M. Gottman and Nan Silver, *The Seven Principles for Making Marriage Work* (New York: Crown, 1999). *69 percent of these happy couples* Ibid. *comes with the territory"* Personal interview. *Solve problems as a team* The tips in this and the following paragraphs are drawn from my eight years as a relationship writer for *New Woman* magazine and thirty-plus years of happy marriage. *"ventilation theory" ... disproved* For a full discussion, see Carol Tavris, *Anger: The Misunderstood Emotion* (New York: Simon & Schuster, 1989). *"remarkable healing powers"* Richard Fitzgibbons, "Anger and the Healing Power of Forgiveness: A Psychiatrist's View," in Robert D. Enright and Joanna North, eds., *Exploring Forgiveness* (Madison: University of Wisconsin Press, 1998), 63–74.

Chapter 13: Losing Two Kinds of Binge-Eating Fat

25 to 30 percent who attend ... clinics R. L. Spitzer et al., "Binge Eating Disorder: A Multisite Field Trial of the Diagnostic Criteria," *International Journal of Eating Disorders* 11 (1992): 191–203; and R. L. Spitzer et al., "Binge Eating Disorder: Its Further Validation in a Multisite Study," *International Journal of Eating Disorders* 13 (Mar. 1993): 137–53. *Christopher G. Fairburn* From his book *Overcoming Binge Eating* (New York: Guilford, 1995). Most of the information in the two paragraphs following is also from Fairburn. *one Columbia University study* J. A. Goldfein et al., "Eating Behavior in Binge-Eating Disorder," *International Journal of Eating Disorders* 14, no. 4 (Dec. 1993): 427–31.   *Some female runners* Dr. Judith Rodin, *Body Traps* (New York: Morrow, 1991), 214.   *debting* Fairburn, *Overcoming Binge Eating*, 54.   *Bulimia Nervosa (BN) ... Binge-Eating Disorder (BED)* The distinctions between BN and BED are described in a number of places, including Fairburn; B. Timothy Walsh and Michael J. Devlin, "Eating Disorders: Progress and Problems," *Science* 280 (May 29, 1998): 1387–90; and Susan Z. Yanovski, "Obesity and Eating Disorders," in Bray et al., eds. *Handbook of Obesity.*   *"tension" as a binge trigger ... drinking alcohol* S. F. Abraham and P. J. V. Beumont, "How Patients Describe Bulimia and Binge Eating," *Psychological Medicine* 12 (1982): 625–35.   *trigger in terms of a pattern* Johan Vanderlinden and Walter Vandereycken, *Trauma, Dissociation, and Impulse Dyscontrol in Eating Disorders* (New York: Brunner/Mazel, 1997), 98.   *young women currently on diets* G. C. Patton et al., "Abnormal Eating Attitudes in London Schoolgirls—A Prospective Epidemiological Study: Outcome at Twelve Month Follow-up," *Psychological Medicine* 20, no. 2 (May 1990): 383–94.   *90 percent success rate* See Fairburn's book *Overcoming Binge Eating.*   *chocolate contains antioxidants* A. L. Waterhouse et al., "Antioxidants in Chocolate," *Lancet* 348, no. 9030 (Sept. 1996): 834.   *may combat cancer* C. Sanbongi et al., "Polyphenols in Chocolate, Which Have Antioxidant Activity, Modulate Immune Functions in Humans in Vitro," *Cellular Immunology* 177, no. 2 (May 1, 1997): 129–36.   *famous aerialist Karl Wallenda* Warren Bennis and Burt Nanus, *Leaders: The Strategies for Taking Charge* (New York: Harper & Row, 1985), 70.   *"the miracle question"* This technique is fully described in Barbara McFarland's book *Brief Therapy and Eating Disorders* (San Francisco: Jossey-Bass, 1995).   *woman who eventually became a winner* Ibid., 109–10.   *another woman who eventually beat her binge eating* Ibid., 115.   *49 percent ... grew up in families with alcohol or drug abuse* Susan Z. Yanovski et al., "Association of Binge Eating Disorder and Psychiatric Comorbidity in Obese Subjects," *American Journal of Psychiatry* 150 (Oct. 10, 1993): 1472–79.   *framework of success rather than failure* Lindsey Hall and Leigh Cohn, eds., *Beating Bulimia: What Has Worked for Me/By 217 Recovered and Recovering Bulimics* (Santa Barbara, Calif.: Gurze Books, 1984). Subsequent quotes from winners are also from Hall and Cohn.

Chapter 14: Losing Polycystic Ovary Fat

10 percent of women ... vast majority don't know it Florence P. Haseltine et al., "Proceedings of a Symposium: An NICHD Conference: Androgens and Women's Health," *American Journal of Medicine* 98 (Jan. 26, 1995): 1A–1S.   *50 to 80 percent ... are overweight* Robert A. Wild, "Obesity, Lipids, Cardiovascular Risk, and Androgen Excess," *American Journal of Medicine* 98 (Jan. 16, 1995): 1A-27S–1A-32S.   *two types of PCOS* J. L. Cresswell et al., "Fetal Growth, Length of Gestation, and Polycystic Ovaries in Adult Life," *Lancet* 350, no. 9085 (Oct. 18, 1997): 1131–35.   *unwanted body hair ... in 60 percent of overweight women* G. S. Conway et al., "Heterogeneity of the Polycystic Ovary Syndrome: Clinical, Endocrine and Ultrasound Features in 556 Patients," *Clinical Endocrinology* 30 (1989): 459–70.   *more overweight ... the more likely you are to have this problem* D. J. Evans et al., "Body Fat Typography in Women with Androgen Excess," *International Journal of Obesity* 12 (1988): 157–62.   *study of sixty-one British families* W. M. Hague et al., "Familial Polycystic Ovaries: A Genetic Disease?" *Clinical Endocrinology* 29 (Dec. 1988): 593–605.   *premature baldness in men* D. Ferriman and A. W. Purdie, "The Inheritance of Polycystic Ovarian Disease and Possible Relationship to Premature Balding," *Clinical Endocrinology* 11 (Sept. 1979): 291–99. Also, A. H. Carey et al., "Evidence for a Single Gene Effect in Polycystic Ovaries and Male Pattern Baldness," *Clinical Endocrinology* 38 (1993): 653–58.   *87 percent ... versus 47 percent* Richard S. Legro, "The Genetics of Polycystic Ovary Syndrome," *American Journal of Medicine* 98 (Jan. 16, 1995): 1A-9S–1A-16S.   *ten times that amount* Geoffrey Redmond, M.D., *The Good News about Women's Hormones* (New York: Warner, 1995), 37.   *highest testosterone levels also weighed the most* Conway et al., "Heterogeneity."   *diabetes in your twenties or thirties* Andrea Dunaif, "Insulin Resistance and Ovarian Dysfunction," in David E. Moller, ed., *Insulin Resistance* (New York: Wiley, 1993).   *Swedish study found* E. Dahlgren et al., "Polycystic Ovary Syndrome and Risk for Myocardial Infarction," *Acta Obstetrica Gynecologica Scandinavia* 71 (1992): 599–604.   *22 and 33 percent ... ovaries that appear polycystic* Adam Balen, "Pathogenesis of Polycystic Ovary Syndrome—The Enigma Unravels?" *Lancet* 354 (Sept. 18, 1999): 966–67.   *Testosterone ... lowest in mid-afternoon* Redmond, *The Good News*, 205–7.   *University of Gothenburg study* Goran Cullberg et al., "Effects of a Low-Dose Desogestrel-Ethinylestradiol, Combination on Hirsuitism, Androgens, and Sex Hormone Binding Globulin in Women with a Polycystic Ovary Syndrome," *Acta Obstetrica Gynecologica Scandinavia* 64 (1985): 195–202.   *the New England Journal of Medicine* Robert DeFronzo et al., "Efficacy of Metformin in Patients with Non-Insulin-Dependent Diabetes Mellitus," *New England Journal of Medicine* (Aug. 31, 1995): 541–49.   *A number of smaller studies* See, for example, E. M., Velazquez et al., "Menstrual Cyclicity after Metformin Therapy in Polycystic Ovary Syndrome," *Obstetrics and Gynecology* 90 (Sept. 1997): 392–95; E. M. Velazquez et al., "Metformin Therapy Is Associated with a Decrease in Plasma Plasminogen Activator Inhibitor-1, Lipoprotein(a), and Immunoreactive Insulin Levels in Patients with the Polycystic Ovary Syndrome," *Metabolism* 4 (April 1997): 454–57.   *A few women lose 50, 60, or 70 pounds* Charles Glueck, personal interview.   *in the blood, called lactic acidosis* Jean D. Lalau et al., "Role of Metformin Accumulation in Metformin-Associated Lactic Acidosis," *Diabetes Care* 18 (June 1995): 779–84.   *If ten million took it for two years* DeFronzo, "Efficacy of Metformin."   *Fructus lycii ... lowered cholesterol ... and triglycerides* Y. Guan and S. Zhao, "Yishou Jiangzhi (de-blood-lipid) Tablets in the Treatment of Hyperlipemia," *Journal of Traditional Chinese Medicine* 3 (Sept. 1995): 178–79.   *Fructus lycii "protected" DNA in such a way this herb may "play an important role in preventing cancer"* D.S. Xu T.Q. Kong, and J.Q. Ma, "The Inhibitory Effect of Extracts from *Fructus lycii* and *Rhizoma polygonati* on in Vitro DNA Breakage by Alternariol," *Biomedical and Environmental Sciences* 9 (Mar. 1996): 67–70.   *"the sovereign herb"* Harriet Beinfield and Efrem Korngold, *Between Heaven and Earth* (New York: Ballantine, 1991) 276.   *Andrew Weil, M.D.* Andrew Weil, *Spontaneous Healing* (New York: Knopf, 1995), 181.

Chapter 15: Losing Night-Eating Fat

NES was first observed Albert J. Stunkard et al., "The Night-Eating Syndrome," *American Journal of Medicine* 19 (1955): 78–86.   *About 10 percent of overweight women* University of Pennsylvania press release, "Night Eating Syndrome," August 17, 1999.   *27 percent of seriously overweight* Colleen S. W. Rand et al., "The Night Eating Syndrome in the General Population and among Postoperative Obesity Surgery Patients," *International Journal of Eating Disorders* 22 (1997): 65–69.   *eight students ... deprived of rapid eye movement (REM)* I reported this finding in "Diet Traps," *Woman's Day*, April 12, 1996.   *sleep deprivation usually leads to an increased consumption of more than 10 to 15 percent* Ibid.   *study conducted jointly* Grethe Stoa Birketvedt et al., "Behavioral and Neuroendocrine Characteristics of the Night-Eating Syndrome," *JAMA* 282, no. 7 (Aug. 18, 1999): 657–63.   *William C. Dement* Personal interview.   *With NES, leptin levels stay low* Birketvedt, "Behavioral and Neuroendocrine Characteristics."   *Melatonin is the hormone.* From William Dement's *The Promise of Sleep* (New York: Dell, 1999).   *NES sufferers, melotonin is much lower* Birketvedt, "Behavioral and Neuroendocrine Characteristics."   *"premenstrual insomnia"* This and the rest of this paragraph come from Dement, *The Promise of Sleep.*   *some caffeine left in your system at 11 P.M.* Ibid.   *Insomnia promoters include* Check the side effects of these or any other drugs you may be taking in the *Physicians' Desk Reference* at your local library.   *bright light early ... Bright light later* Sonia Ancoli-Israel, director of the sleep-disorders clinic at the VA Hospital Medical Center in San Diego, personal interview.   *At least half of insomniacs* Dement, *The Promise of Sleep*, 136.   *trained athletes spend more time in the deep, restful stages of sleep* James Horne, "Human Slow Wave Sleep: A Review and Appraisal of Recent Findings, with Implications for Sleep Functions, and Psychiatric Illness," *Experientia* 48 no. 10 (Oct. 15, 1992): 941–54.   *Alcohol also has paradoxical effect* Dement, *The Promise of Sleep.*   *75 percent of recovering alcoholic women* Colleen S.W. Rand et al., "Patterns of food and alcohol consumption in a group of bulimic women," *Bulletin of the Society of Psychologists in Addictive Behaviors* (now *Psychology of Addictive Behaviors*) 5 (1986): 95–104.   *Even a bright bathroom light at 2 A.M.* Ancoli-Israel interview.

Chapter 16: Losing Post-Pregnancy Fat

In one Swedish study Stephan Rossner, "Weight Gain in Pregnancy," *Human Reproduction* 12, Suppl. 1 (1997): 110–15.   *Alan Stein and coworkers* Alan Stein et al., "Eating Habits and Attitudes in the Postpartum Period," *Psychosmatic Medicine* 58 (1996): 321–25.   *70 percent of new mothers . . . 39 percent are still unhappy* Debra Tooke Crowell, "Weight Change in the Post Partum Period," Journal of Nurse-Midwifery 40, no. 5 (Sept./Oct. 1995): 418–23. This is a good, readable review of the literature on pregnancy and weight gain.   *Then the theory changed* For a good review of pregnancy weight literature, see Lorraine O. Walker, "Weight Gain after Childbirth: A Women's Health Concern?" *Annals of Behavioral Medicine* 17, no. 2 (1995): 132–41.   *current advised weight gains* From the Institute of Medicine, National Academy of Sciences.   *clinic at St. Luke's–Roosevelt Hospital* Sally Ann Lederman et al., "Body Fat and Water Changes during Pregnancy in Women with Different Body Weight and Weight Gain," *Obstetrics & Gynecology* 90, no. 4, part 1 (Oct. 1997): 483–88.   *no relationship between exercise and weight loss* C. W. Schauberger et al., "Factors That Influence Weight Loss in the Puerperium," *Obstetrics & Gynecology* 79 (Mar. 1992): 424–29.   *University of Pennsylvania* Karen Morin et al., "Nutrition and Exercise in Overweight and Obese Postpartum Women," *Applied Nursing Research* 12, no. 1 (Feb. 1999): 13–21.   *women who bottle-fed lost more weight* D. Manning-Dalton and L. H. Allen, "The Effects of Lactation on Energy and Protein Consumption, Postpartum Weight Change, and Body Composition of Well-Nourished North American Women," *Nutritional Research* 3 (1983): 293–308; M. M. Brewer et al., "Postpartum Changes in Maternal Weight and Body Fat Depots in Lactating vs. Non-Lactating Women," *American Journal of Clinical Nutrition* 49 (1989): 259–65.   *Go with the flow* Much of my understanding of systems for this and the subsequent section came from my experience of writing a book about childrearing with University of Connecticut biopsychologist Evelyn B. Thoman.   *postpartum thyroiditis* Material for this section came from J. H. Lazarus, "Clinical Manifestations of Postpartum Thyroid Disease," *Thyroid* 9, no. 7 (July 1999): 685–89; C. R. Fantz et al., "Thyroid Function During Pregnancy," *Clinical Chemistry* 45, no. 12 (Dec. 1999): 2250–58; D. Glinoer, "What Happens to the Normal Thyroid during Pregnancy?" *Thyroid* 9, no. 7 (July, 1999): 631–35.   *women . . . most dissatisfied with their bodies* Helen E. Harris et al., "Relative Importance of Heritable Characteristics and Lifestyle in the Development of Maternal Obesity," *Journal of Epidemiology and Community Health* 53 (1999): 66–74.   *developed full-blown eating disorders* Stein et al., "Eating Habits."   *In truth, only 28 percent* L. C. Olsen and M. H. Mundt, "Postpartum Weight Loss in a Nurse-Midwifery Practice, *Journal of Nurse-Midwifery* 31 (1986): 177–81.   *Operating Instructions* Anne Lamott, *Operating Instructions* (New York: Fawcett, 1994).   *A Duke University study suggests* Linda J. Luecken et al., "Stress in Employed Women: Impact of Marital Status and Children at Home on Neurohormone Output and Home Strain," *Psychosomatic Medicine* 59 (1997): 352–59.   *still haven't turned over the vigilance* Kathleen C. Light, "Stress in Employed Women: A Woman's Work Is Never Done If She's a Working Mom" (editorial), *Psychosomatic Medicine* 59 (1997): 360–61.   *fathers' effort hormones go down . . . women's effort hormones . . . go up* Marianne Frankenhaeuser et al., "Stress On and Off the Job as Related to Sex and Occupational Status in White-Collar Workers," *Journal of Organizational Behavior* 10 (1989): 321–46.   *half the women in a survey* A. Cassidy, "What Pushes Your Stress Button?" *Working Mother,* July/August, 1996, 18–22.   *Women who develop the blues have . . . higher cortisol levels* T. Okano and J. Nomura, "Endocrine Study of Maternity Blues," *Progress in Neuropsychopharmcol Biol Psychiatry* 16, no. 6 (1992): 921–32.   *feeling unsupported by a spouse* T. S. Brugha et al., "The Leicester 500 Project: Social Support and the Development of Postnatal Depressive Symptoms, a Prospective Cohort Study," *Psychological Medicine* 28, no. 7 (Jan. 1998): 63–79; also Lorraine O. Walker, "Weight and Weight-Related

Distress after Childbirth: Relationships to Stress, Social Support, and Depressive Symptoms," *Journal of Holistic Nursing* 15, no. 4 (Dec. 1997): 389–405.   *powerful predictor of the blues was a sense of "pessimism"* J. T. Condon and T. L. Watson, "The Maternity Blues: Exploration of a Psychological Hypothesis," *Acta Psychiatriatrica Scandinavia* 76, no. 2 (Aug. 1987): 164–71. *a woman who gained 150 pounds* P. J. Bradley, "Does Pregnancy Cause Obesity?" *Medical Journal of Australia* 151 (1989): 543–44.   *44 percent of first-time mothers over age 35* Michael Prysak et al., "Pregnancy Outcome in Nulliparous Women 35 Years and Older," *Obstetrics & Gynecology* 85 (Jan. 1995): 65–70.   *Swedish women had many PTSD symptoms* E. L. Ryding et al., "Post-traumatic Stress Reactions after Emergency Cesarean Section," *Acta Obstet Gynecol Scand* 76, no. 9 (Oct. 1997): 856–61.   *33 percent of women* Ibid.   *55 percent of C-Section mothers reported fearing for their own lives* E. L. Ryding et al., "Experiences of Emergency Cesarean Section: A Phenomenological Study of 53 Women," *Birth* 25, no. 4 (Dec. 1998): 246–51.   *doctor with a high-risk practice ... low-risk practice* Sidney M. Wolfe, M.D., *Women's Health Alert* (Reading, Mass.: Addison-Wesley, 1991) 95–96.

Chapter 17: Losing Medication-Caused Fat

tricyclic antidepressants ... cause weight gain in 89 percent Madelyn H. Fernstrom and David J. Kupfer, "Antidepressant-Induced Weight Gain: A Comparison Study of Four Medications," *Psychiatry Research* 26 (Oct. 10, 1988): 265–71.   *More than 50 million prescriptions* Marc Kaufman, "Newer Antidepressants Not Better, Study Says; Federal Analysis Suggests Fewer Side Effects Drive Popularity of Prozac and Similar Drugs," *Washington Post*, April 6, 1999, p. Z07.   *28 percent of patients taking ... amitriptyline* Fernstrom and Kupfer, "Antidepressant-Induced Weight Gain."   *Breast cancer patients ... gain weight* Pamela J. Goodwin et al., "Weight Gain in Women with Localized Breast Cancer—a Descriptive Study," *Breast Cancer Research and Treatment* 11 (1988): 59–66. For more information on breast cancer treatment–linked weight gains, see Chapter 17, "Losing Medication-Caused Fat."   *one international study* Jerilynn Prior et al., "Premenopausal Ovariectomy-Related Bone Loss: A Randomized, Double-Blind, One-Year Trial of Conjugated Estrogen or Medroxyprogesterone Acetate," *Journal of Bone and Mineral Research* 12 (Nov. 11, 1997): 1851–63.   *Maine Women's Health Study* Karen J. Carlson et al., "The Maine Women's Health Study I: Outcomes of Hysterectomy," *Obsterics & Gynecology* 83 (1994): 556–65. The authors claim that if women didn't have post-hysterectomy weight problems at both six months *and* twelve months after surgery, weight wasn't really a "problem." They then go on to maintain that only 12 percent of women struggled with post-hysterectomy fat. But this is faulty thinking, because women who began gaining weight after the surgery may not have defined it as a "problem" at six months (when they may have gained only a few pounds), but may have seen it as a real problem by twelve months (when they'd gained more). It's also possible that some women's ovaries stopped working during the subsequent year, and they then developed weight problems as a result.   *Nora Coffey* Personal interview.   *about 100 calories a day* E.T. Poehlman et al., "Changes in Energy Balance and Body Composition in Menopause: a Controlled Longitudinal Study," *Annals of Internal Medicine* 123, no. 9 (Nov. 1, 1995): 673–75.   *ovary removal in rats ... alters levels of leptin* Shu-Chen Shu et al., "Fluctuation of Serum Leptin Level in Rats after Ovariectomy and the Influence of Estrogen Supplement," *Life Sciences* 64, no. 24 (1999): 2299–2306.   *one Finnish study* R. Luoto et al., "Cardiovascular Morbidity in Relation to Ovarian Function after Hysterectomy," *Obstetrics & Gynecology* 85, no. 4. (April 1995): 515–22.   *women with the least schooling were ... 15 times* Diana Kuh and Susan Stirling, "Sociological Variations in Admissions for Disease of Female Genital System and Breast in a National Cohort Aged 15–43," *British Medical Journal* 311 (Sept. 30, 1995): 840–43.   *high school dropouts also have this surgery* K. Kjerulff et al., "The Socioeconomic Correlates of Hysterectomies in the United States," *American Journal of Public Health* 83, no. 1 (Jan. 1993): 106–8.   *UCLA researchers surveyed 109 drug ads* M. S. Wilkes et al., "Pharmaceutical Advertisements in Leading Medical Journals: Experts' Assessments," *Annals of Internal Medicine* 116, no. 11 (June 1, 1992): 912–19.   *trips to ritzy resorts* J. P. Orlowski and L. Wateska, "The Effects of Pharmaceutical Firm Enticements on Physician Prescribing Patterns.) There's No Such Thing as a Free Lunch," *Chest* 102, no. 1 (July 1992): 270–73.   *Physician's Desk Reference (PDR)* This is the source of nearly all of the drug information in this chapter.   *Eric P. Cohen, M.D.* Personal interview.   *$600 million a year* This figure is several years old, and the amount is probably higher by now.   *Consumer Reports survey* Appeared in June 1996.   *Steffie Woolhandler, M.D.* Personal interview.

Chapter 18: Losing Post-Trauma Fat

25 percent of women For a good review of all the trauma literature, including incidence, see Judith Herman, *Trauma and Recovery* (New York; BasicBooks, 1997).   *study at Brown University* Teresa K. King et al., "History of Sexual Abuse and Obesity Treatment Outcome," *Addictive Behaviors* 21, no. 3 (1996): 283–90.   *most common symptoms* Bessel A. van der Kolk et al., "Dissociation, Somatization, and Affect Dysregulation: The Complexity of Adaptation to Trauma," *American Journal of Psychiatry* 153, no. 7 (July 1996): 83–93. See also Herman, *Trauma and Recovery*, and Aphrodite Matsakis, *Post-Traumatic Stress Disorder: A Complete Treatment Guide* (Oakland, Calif.: New Harbinger, 1994)   *66.5 percent of women at one gastrointestinal clinic* Jane Lesserman et al., "Sexual and Physical Abuse History in Gastroenterology Practice: How Types of Abuse Impact Health Status," *Psychosomatic Medicine* 58 (1996): 4–15.   *38 percent of women in one study didn't* L. M. Williams, "Recall of Childhood Trauma: A Prospective Study of Women's Memories of Childhood Sexual Abuse," *Journal of Consulting Clinical Psychology* 62, no. 6 (Dec. 1994): 1167–76.   *"the body keeps the score"* B. A. van der Kolk, "The Body Keeps the Score: Approaches to the Psychobiology of Posttraumatic Stress Disorder," in B. A. van der Kolk et al., eds., *Traumatic Stress: The Effects of Overwhelming Experience on Mind, Body, and Society* (New York: Guilford, 1996), 214–41.   *deregulates the cortisol highway* See, for example, Rachel Yehuda et al., "Hypothalamic-Pituitary-Adrenal Dysfunction in Posttraumatic Stress Disorder," *Biological Psychiatry* 30 (1991): 1031–48.   *emotionally "hijacking"* Daniel Goleman, *Emotional Intelligence* (New York: Bantam, 1995).   *fifty-five Turkish activists* Metin Basoglu et al., "Psychological Effects of Torture: A Comparison of Tortured with Nontortured Political Activists in Turkey," *American Journal of Psychiatry* 151, no. 1 (Jan. 1994): 76–81.   *"the subjects in our own quests for the truth"* Judith Herman, *Trauma and Recovery*.

Chapter 19: Designing Your Superconfidence Diet

50 percent of the variations in our cholesterol levels are genetically determined Artemis P. Simopoulos, "Genetic Variation and Nutrition," *Nutrition Today* 30, no. 4 (July/Aug. 1995): 157–67.   *30 to 60 percent of the variations in our blood pressure* J. G. Mongeau, "Heredity and Blood Pressure," *Semin Nephrology* 9 (1989): 208–16.   *an Australian study* N. A. Morrison et al., "Prediction of Bone Density from Vitamin D Receptor Alleles," *Nature* 367 (1994): 284–87.   *Black people . . . more likely . . . salt-sensitive* M. Rowland and J. Roberts, "Blood Pressure Levels and Hypertension in Persons Ages 6–74 Years; United States, 1976–80," *Advance Data* 8, no. 84 (Oct. 8, 1982): 1–11.   *"gluten-sensitive" people* Simopoulos, "Genetic Variation and Nutrition."   *7 to 16 percent of Eskimos* Ibid.   *the "sugar/fat seesaw"* John E. Blundell and Neil A. King, "Overconsumption as a Cause of Weight Gain: Behavioral-Physiological Interactions in the Control of Food Intake (Appetite)," *The Origins and Consequences of Obesity* (Chichester: Wiley, 1996), 138–58.   *led to an increase of 11 percent* D. J. Naismith and C. Rhodes, "Adjustments in Energy Intake Following the Covert Removal of Sugar from the Diet," *Journal of Human Nutrition and Dietetics* 8 (1995), 167–75.   *the Nurses' Health Study* G. A. Colditz et al., "Patterns of Weight Change and Their Relation to Diet in a Cohort of Healthy Women," *American Journal of Clinical Nutrition* 51 (1990), 1100–1105.   *83 percent of Asians flushed* Simopoulos, "Genetic Variation and Nutrition."   *Cardiologist Dean Ornish* Dr. Dean Ornish's *Program for Reversing Heart Disease* (New York: Ivy Books, 1996).   *one study reported in the* International Journal of Obesity, Berit L. Heitmann et al., "Does Dietary Fat Promote Weight Gain in Genetically Predisposed Individuals? A Prospective Study of Swedish Women," *Inter-*

national Journal of Obesity 17, Suppl. 2 (1993), 108. The finding that fat makes only genetically predisposed women fat was more fully reported in Berit Heitmann et al., "Dietary Fat Intake and Weight Gain in Women Genetically Predisposed for Obesity," *American Journal of Clinical Nutrition* 61 (1995), 1213–17.   *Lawrence Berkeley National Laboratory (LBNL)* Personal interview. I originally reported this in *Reader's Digest New Choices*.   *trans-fats deliver a double whammy* A. Ascherio et al., "Trans Fatty Acids and Coronary Heart Disease," *New England Journal of Medicine* 340, no. 25 (June 24, 1999): 1994–98.   *a French study reported in* Circulation M. de Lorgeril et al., "Mediterranean Diet, Traditional Risk Factors, and the Rate of Cardiovascular Complications after Myocardial Infarction: Final Report of the Lyon Diet Heart Study," *Circulation* 99, no. 6 (Feb. 16. 1999): 779–85.   *more recent research in Europe* B. L. Heitmann, L. Lissner, et al., "Dietary Fat Intake and Weight Gain in Women Genetically Predisposed for Obesity," *American Journal of Clinical Nutrition* 61, no. 6 (June 1995):1213–17.   *only in sedentary women* L. Lissner et al., "Low-Fat Diets May Prevent Weight Gain in Sedentary Women: Prospective Observations from the Population Study of Women in Gothenburg, Sweden," *Obesity Research* 5, no. 1 (Jan. 1997): 43–48.   *baffling experiment* Alan R. Hirsch and R. Gomez, "Weight Reduction through Inhalation of Odorants," *Journal of Neurological and Orthopedic Medicine and Surgery* 16 (1995): 26–31.

Chapter 20: Becoming an Exercise Winner
This chapter is based largely on my personal experience as an exercise winner, coupled with my interviews with exercise winners. Several points in this chapter were previously reported in my articles in *Reader's Digest* ("Don't Be an Exercise Dropout," Aug. 1991) and *Woman's Day* ("Get Up and Go!" Oct. 3, 1998).

Acknowledgments

One of the great pleasures of writing a book is not only getting to work closely with old friends but also getting to meet so many wonderful new people. First of all, a warm thank-you goes out to the winners who invented ways to control their weight and shared their enlightenment with me. Even before anyone told them *why*, they learned *how*. A special thanks also goes out to C. Wayne Callaway for being so generous with his time and dropping out of the professional mode long enough to explain to me the "something extra" that really got this book rolling. Others without whom this book could never have been written include those questing scientists who care so passionately about the truth that they're willing to go to "war" over it: especially Adam Drewnowski, Reubin Andres, Susan Yanovski, George Blackburn, Gerald Reaven, George Bray, Susan Wooley, and countless others too numerous to mention. A special thanks goes out to the three key scientists whose work forms the backbone of this book.

First, to Swedish endocrinologist Per Bjorntorp, M.D., head of the Department of Heart and Lung Diseases at the University of Gothenburg's Sahlgren's Hospital in Gothenburg, Sweden. Plug his name into the National Library of Medicine's online library of major medical journals, and you'll retrieve hundreds of citations for articles he has either authored or coauthored since 1965. For years, he has been asking the question: How are ancient humans adapting to our stress-filled, fast-paced modern age? The answer: we're getting fat. In the 1,012-page *Handbook of Obesity*, a $245 textbook for physicians-in-training coedited by George Bray and usually found only in university medical libraries, Bjorntorp wrote the chapter describing how visceral fat develops. As you now know, it almost always starts with a powerless or "defeat" reaction to stress, accompanied by "stress-reducing" habits like smoking, drinking alcohol, and exercising too little. No one understands the new paradigm shift in obesity research better than Bjorntorp, who graciously read large parts of the manuscript for accuracy.

Second, my appreciation goes out to Marianne Frankenhaeuser, Ph.D., the brilliant Swedish psychoendocrinologist who was the first to verify and clearly describe how our two *separate and independent* stress systems work and was kind enough to read an early draft of my descriptions of her work. Interested in how "ancient humans" were adapting to modern technology with its information overload, increasing time pressure, and fast-paced living, Frankenhaeuser garnered a grant from the Swedish Medical Research Council and used it to start a psychology department at Stockholm University. Then she began watching people under different kinds of stress to see how they reacted. She was the first to clearly demonstrate that catecholamines and cortisol (the same hormones that dissolve and store fat) are, respectively, the effort hormones and the distress hormone. Her work provides one of the strongest and most crucial links in the new understanding of stress and its effects on the body.

The third paradigm shifter without whose work this book could not have been written is Albert Bandura, Ph.D., professor of social sciences in psychology at Stanford University and past president of the American Psychological Association. The father of self-efficacy theory, the study of how people take charge (or choose *not* to take charge), Bandura's influential research has sparked research around the world, including more than two thousand studies on Medline alone. He has been elected to the American Academy of Arts and Sciences and the Institute of Medicine of the National Academy of Sciences and has received honorary degrees from eleven universities. It was his self-efficacy theory and the studies of how self-efficacy affects weight control that led me to find the weight-loss winners.

Many other researchers also generously shared their time and expertise, including Claude Bouchard, Vincent Felitti, Redford Williams, Delia Smith, William Castelli, Robert Jeffrey, Randy Seeley, Lorraine O. Walker, Ridha Arem, Aaron Folsom, Andrea Dunaif, and more.

On a more personal level, I'm indebted to my three favorite magazine editors, Elena Serocki at the *Reader's Digest*, Nissa Simon at *New Choices*, and Stephanie Abarbanel at *Woman's Day*, for giving me a "leave of absence" to write this book and welcoming me back with such enthusiasm when it was over.

My gratitude also goes out to my inveterate researcher, Erin Browder, for her hard work and diligence, as she pored through the medical journals and gleaned so much information from the Stanford University Medical Library. At crucial moments, she found important studies that opened new doors to my understanding.

Thank you also to my agent, Suzanne Gluck, who kept the book on course from the beginning and shepherded it to the wonderful team at Wiley: especially my ever-supportive, ever-patient editor Tom Miller, a master of structure; marketers extraordinaire Kitt Allan and Laura Cusack; senior editor Carole Hall; publisher Gerry Helferich; associate managing editor Sibylle Kazeroid; and copy editor Alexa Selph. Thanks also to Karen Gerwin at ICM for diligently pursuing magazine sales.

Finally, I wish to thank Dustin Browder and Jen Browder, whose supportive conversations were a welcome respite from the otherwise relentless research and writing that occupied more than one solid year of my life. Last, but far from least, a heartfelt thank-you beyond words to my husband and writing collaborator, Walter, whose support and love remained ever constant through a process that was at once one of the most exhausting and exhilarating of my life.

Index